MY LIFE AND WORK WITH ALFRED VOGEL

My Life and Work with Alfred Vogel

An autobiography packed with expert advice for healthy living

Jan de Vries

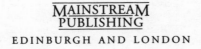
MAINSTREAM
PUBLISHING
EDINBURGH AND LONDON

First published in Great Britain in 2005 by
MAINSTREAM PUBLISHING COMPANY (EDINBURGH) LTD
7 Albany Street
Edinburgh EH1 3UG

ISBN 1 84018 985 1

A catalogue record for this book
is available from the British Library

Typeset in Caslon

Printed and bound in Great Britain by
William Clowes Ltd, Beccles, Suffolk

Contents

Preface

The first time I actually came face to face with the late Alfred Vogel was in 1958, just after I graduated in pharmacy, when, by chance, I sat next to him at a lecture in Amsterdam. I did not know who he was at that time but when he started up a conversation and enthused about his work, I was almost instantaneously converted to his way of thinking.

I was so fascinated by all he said that I travelled to Switzerland to see what he was doing there and we talked about the prospect of opening the first naturopathic clinic in Holland. As we discussed the future of medicine and health, we came to the conclusion that by making such a clinic accessible to those searching for an alternative approach to orthodox medicine we would be taking a step in the right direction.

Roode Wald, which opened in 1959, developed into one of the finest clinics I have ever known. In the first volume of my autobiography, *A Step at a Time*, I have written of the many memories I have of the years spent there and how during that time the working relationship between Alfred Vogel and me developed into a deep, lasting friendship.

The clinic ran successfully for a number of years but,

eventually, due to a number of factors, including the lack of support from the government and staffing problems, we were forced to close it down. Fortunately, however, despite its closure, the valuable remedies that Alfred had created over the years – many of which were his own formulations – continued to be produced so that those in need could still benefit from them. When I think of all the Bioforce remedies available throughout the world today, I know if Alfred could see the results of his hard work and pioneering activities, he would be very happy.

Alfred realised early on that he had one mission in life and that was basically to help people. He also told me that the most important thing that one can do in life is to share one's knowledge with others and I am pleased to say that his influence continues to be felt today. We worked together for nearly 40 years off and on, and, although we often went our separate ways, we regularly met up to discuss health issues. I feel privileged that I was the only pupil to whom he taught everything he knew about health and healthy living. He instilled in me that same great desire to help others and every day I feel proud that I have been able to carry on in his footsteps.

Alfred's interest in learning all about plants and herbs started at a very early age. While he was still a young boy, his mother and grandmother shared with him their knowledge about the benefits of herbal medicines. Then, between 1920 and 1932, he managed a health food store in Basel and it was here that he met his wife Sophie. He decided to expand on his knowledge by studying homoeopathy, naturopathy and botany, and by his late 20s, he had turned his property in Teufen into a residential clinic. Beside the clinic, he worked in the fields tending his plants and herbs, which he greatly loved.

He visited various colleges and universities with the aim of learning as much as he could, and through his lifelong devotion became, in my opinion, probably the greatest botanist of all time. He would meet people from all corners of the world and was eager to compare his thoughts and findings with others. He was very open minded and was always willing to listen to other people's ideas.

Sadly, however, his amazing findings were not always appreciated, as the Swiss are a very conservative nation. At the start of his career, as he tried to secure acceptance for his unorthodox methods, it soon became clear that a mammoth task lay before him. But despite apparent resistance to his ideas, he continued with his efforts.

Alfred never advertised his services but his reputation grew rapidly by word of mouth and, eventually, he became known to people all over the world. As his business grew, he was able to employ more qualified staff, including doctors. In 1929, he published his first monthly magazine, *Das Neue Leben* (New Life) – renamed *Gesundheits Nachrichten* (Health News) in 1944 – in which he shared an insight into his work with his readers.

As he was always totally engrossed in what he was doing, he could be quite intolerant of distractions. I had personal experience of this when I first arrived in Teufen to meet him and found him working in the fields. He was so absorbed in his plants and herbs that I was given a cold reception and instructed to come back later. When he had finished work, he met me in the little boardroom in his clinic and the atmosphere between us quickly changed: from that moment on, we were the greatest of friends. I often think back to that meeting, when he trusted me enough to tell me about many of his findings. Eventually, he would even give me control of the recipes that he had painstakingly formulated over many years.

In the Foreword that he wrote for my book *Traditional Home & Herbal Remedies* ten years before his death in 1996, it becomes clear what our friendship meant to him. It is for that reason I have decided to repeat that Foreword in this book. It also explains a lot about his work and shows how he devoted his life to helping to alleviate human suffering.

Jan de Vries

Foreword

This Foreword originally appeared in Traditional Home and Herbal Remedies *in 1986.*

It was a fortunate occasion when I met Jan de Vries in the Netherlands. With pleasure and conviction I spoke of my 40 years' experience in the field of herbal medicine and my views on diet and nourishment. I soon realised that I had an extremely interested listener who fully appreciated my acquired knowledge of the whole sphere of medical science.

Jan de Vries was not only interested to learn everything about my experiences of when, where and how to collect herbs, and which methods were to be followed, he also insisted on taking part in the actual process of extracting beneficial ingredients. As he was a trained and qualified pharmacist, he was already familiar with the world of plants and herbs, and had considerable knowledge in this field. He accepted an invitation to join our firm, which gave us the chance to establish a working relationship which has lasted for years. He was one of my best pupils, if not the very best, and he had the opportunity to further develop his given talents in the field of natural medicine.

I was very happy to share with him my enthusiasm for

nature and the world of plants, as originated by the sovereign power of the Creator. He was also prepared to accept my principle that herbal medicine should always have priority in the treatment of illnesses.

As a result of our experiences, we both agreed that, through knowledge and advice on natural methods and herbal remedies, it was possible to improve one's health and keep illnesses at bay. Nature itself is capable of healing.

Drawing on my many years of experience, I was able to convince Jan de Vries completely that herbal medicine in combination with a natural diet could create positive responses in the body in order to ward off ailments. By creating the right conditions for the body and supplying it with the correct nourishment, one is able to activate one's own regenerative system. In this way it is possible to overcome, as well as cure, ailments. We realise more and more, and my experience over many years in practice has contributed to this, that we don't just have an important role to play in the curing of illnesses but also in the prevention of medical disturbances. This requires us to put emphasis on preventative medicine. Prevention is better than a cure.

This principle plays a major role in our programme. In an effort to clarify this for patients and other interested parties, I myself have written several books, such as *The Nature Doctor: A Manual of Traditional & Complementary Medicine*, *The Liver as the Regulator of our Health* and *Nature: Your Guide to Healthier Living*.

Jan de Vries was immediately prepared to share with his friends, and later with his patients, my experiences and he recommended these books for their information. He is, I am pleased to repeat, my most successful 'pupil'. His success from which many patients have benefited is, however, not only a result of his talents, it is also thanks to the Creator who has supplied so many plants with healing powers.

I am very pleased that Jan de Vries is making the effort to share his knowledge and experiences with us on paper. His books are written in a straightforward manner and can be readily understood by both patients and laymen alike. In them, he deals with natural ways and methods using herbal remedies to overcome ailments and illnesses.

It is important that not just the obvious symptoms are cured, as conventional medicine would teach us. We must look for the cause of the illness in order to continue the treatment and find a cure for the source. Very little benefit is obtained by clearing up an ache or easing a sensitivity if we are not able to eliminate the cause. In order to do this, we should study the whole person and attempt to recognise which factors have contributed to this condition. There could be very many reasons – for example, a breathing difficulty or a movement disorder, shortage of oxygen, rest or sleep. There can be so many causes of a biological imbalance.

Jan de Vries has acquired and developed a large knowledge in this area. With perseverance he builds up an overall picture of total health, not forgetting the physical and mental condition of the patient.

I am convinced that, in this book, he will show many sufferers the right way to recovery in plain and simple language. It is an excellent complement to my books, as we have both sincerely attempted to serve our fellow men and share with them our knowledge acquired from our understanding and experience of the bounty of nature.

Dr Alfred Vogel
1986

Chapter 1

Good health should be treasured and never abused
– for good health leads to happiness.
Alfred Vogel, 1902–96

From reading the Foreword that my great friend Alfred Vogel
wrote for one of my previous books (and which I have repeated
here), it becomes apparent what a wonderful relationship we
had. Vogel and I worked together for over 40 years and I still
believe that he was brought into my young life to give it some
direction – one that I have never regretted. We had very similar
views in that we both wanted to promote good health and we
realised the importance of maintaining a positive mental
attitude, whatever the circumstances might be.

At the time of our first meeting at a lecture on homoeopathy
in Amsterdam in 1958, I was sceptical about the benefits of
complementary therapies. After talking with Vogel, however,
he changed my way of thinking to such a degree that I went to
visit him in Switzerland, where I was so impressed by his work

that I decided to join him. From that date on, my life, like his, has been devoted to alleviating suffering in thousands of people.

He possessed a wonderful spirit. Not only was he a genius but he was also a man with a big heart who cared passionately about his fellow human beings and spent his life striving to achieve good health for everyone. Every single day I treasure the wonderful relationship I had with my great mentor and friend. When my mind is in a quandary, I often think to myself, 'Alfred, what would you do about this?'

The last time I saw him was when I travelled to Zurich just a few weeks before he died. I could see that his condition had deteriorated but he still retained a glimmer of happiness in his eyes as he made humorous remarks about life in general. We chatted together privately for a while, not only reminiscing about the wonderful times of the past but also discussing the present and the future. Although his time was coming to an end, he had an amazingly cheerful attitude and the contented look in his eyes showed that he had led a fulfilling life. Even at that point, he was still offering me advice and ideas.

So who was Alfred Vogel? From the first day we met, when he made such an impression on me, I realised he was a most remarkable, interesting man. He had an unshakeable belief, a great love of nature and a wonderful respect for his Creator.

Alfred was born on 26 October 1902 in a small agricultural village called Aesch near Basel. He was well cared for and his family instilled in him his great love of God and nature. Although he was not an only child, he was a very special individual and this was quickly recognised by his mother and grandmother. These women, who were to play such an important part in his life, were well known in the area for their knowledge of natural remedies and people would often go to them for help and advice. He was particularly influenced by his grandmother, who lived to the ripe old age of 103. Along with his parents, she offered him a lot of practical, sensible advice and put great effort into teaching little Alfred all about nature. His family led a sober life and respected his feelings for the animal and plant worlds; they applauded his vegetarian principles, which they also upheld.

While he was growing up, Alfred wanted to know about everything that was going on around him. Not only did he want to learn as much as he could about the healing properties of plants, he also wanted to research them. This was not always easy and his probing mind often got him into trouble, especially at school, where he sometimes contradicted his teachers. He never accepted anything at face value and would question their reasoning when something did not make sense to him. This was part of his character that drew me to Alfred, as I too was very inquisitive at school.

His enquiring mind also caused the local priest problems when Alfred started to question religion. When he was still young, the local priest said to him, 'Alfredli, do your best in your life, because you will either be a rascal or you will be an extremely good person.' I can certainly testify that he was the latter: he had exceedingly high principles, he always worked hard and he looked for what God had created in nature to help Man. He believed that religion is a personal matter and in order to have a relationship with one's Creator, one has to act from the heart. With that thought in his mind, he felt he had a duty to do everything possible to help his fellow human beings.

When he was younger, his views were quite extreme and not always appreciated by the local Swiss people, who were extremely conventional. Even though Switzerland was neutral during both world wars, Alfred caused controversy with his strong pacifist beliefs. He was a man who loved life and he could not understand why murder and war could be tolerated.

After he left school, Alfred was still eager to learn more about the world around him: indeed, this was part of his character that remained undiminished right till the end. While still in his teens, he visited Maximilian Bircher-Benner's renowned dietary clinic in Zurich. Bircher-Benner was a Swiss physician and a pioneer in nutritional research. At his sanatorium, a balanced diet of raw vegetables and fruit was used as a means to heal patients, and he is also known as the man who invented muesli. Vogel learned a great deal during his time there, and throughout his following career he remained convinced about the importance of food management, especially establishing a balance between protein and carbohydrates, and acidic and alkaline foods.

Following the opening of his first health food store at No. 1 Jurastrasse in 1920, word got around about who Vogel was and it was not long until he had gained a reputation as a great herbalist. As his fame grew, people would consult him when they were not satisfied with the results obtained from their own doctors.

He started to produce a monthly magazine to disseminate information about his findings, and eventually he would write many books. In this, he was fortunate to get some help from a teacher called Sophie – who was later to become his wife. She met Alfred as a customer in his shop and became fascinated by his work. They talked at great length about their mutual interest and grew very close. She also often helped with his lectures and once I got to know her I realised how intelligent and knowledgeable she was in matters relating to herbal medicines and their healing powers.

People came from all over to see Vogel, until his practice expanded to such an extent that he had to move to larger premises. In 1937, he managed to find a suitable place in Teufen, deep in the mountains, where he established his clinic. He became so popular that buses laden with people started to go up the hill to Teufen and it became necessary for people to make appointments well in advance to see this wonderful man. Although he was extremely busy, he always took time to talk and listen to those who were very ill. Doctors would also go to him for guidance and he was never too tired to share his great knowledge whenever possible. Not only did Vogel have time to help the ordinary man in the street but he also made himself available to those who genuinely wanted to study his methods. General Tito of Yugoslavia often asked him for advice and he never failed to help when he could.

I joined Alfred in Teufen to work with him at the clinic and together we achieved a great deal. During his consultations, he started to teach me about what he was doing and he would offer advice whenever possible on how we should treat people. Vogel adhered strictly to the principles of Dr Samuel Hahnemann, the founder of homoeopathy, who argued that Man is not one body but three: physical, mental and emotional. Using holistic methods, these three bodies must be treated together.

It was admirable to see how fervently he researched plants.

Every plant, flower, root and even the bark of a tree has its own signature and characteristic. When we examine them and learn how they grow, they give us a message. Alfred studied as many species as he could and tried to establish whether the signatures of the plants gave an indication about which ailments they might be used to treat. He also needed to guarantee that when prescribing such remedies to patients, they would have no side effects, so a lot of research was involved in preparing his treatments.

It was always a delight to listen to Alfred as he explained the characteristics of different plants. When you step on *Arnica* by mistake, for example, it flops back, telling you that it should be used to treat trauma, while the ingredients of a *Symphytum* root – allantoin, for example – indicate the terrific healing powers of that plant, which is often used to treat wounds and broken bones.

Such was Alfred's relationship with nature that he knew virtually every plant that grew, every flower, every leaf and every bark. His senses were so developed that, even from a distance, he could smell which herbs were growing in a particular area. If he discovered something with which he was unfamiliar, he made every effort to find out about it.

Only the year before he died, I walked with him in the mountains. As he inhaled deeply, he said, 'I can smell wild garlic.' Alfred then went down on his knees and started to scrape at the dirty soil with his bare hands. When he reached the garlic, he pulled out the clean silvery bulb from the ground and not even one speck of dirt had adhered to it. He said, 'Look, even in all that mud and dirt, its silvery-white colour shows us that God gave this to Man to keep his body cleansed.' Alfred knew that garlic is a great antiseptic and should be used to treat viral problems and infections. At the time of writing this book, the newspapers are full of a 'new cure' for the horrific MRSA virus being contracted in hospitals and that 'new cure' is . . . garlic! In fact, Alfred publicised its therapeutic properties as far back as 50 years ago.

Vogel's thirst for knowledge was unquenchable and he was so devoted to learning more from nature that I used to see him working in his herb garden at four or five o'clock in the morning, studying the plants. He often said that we had to dig deep and use the whole plant, thus avoiding the mistake sometimes made by the pharmaceutical industry when they sought a clear pharmacological action from a particular part of a plant or a herb, leading them to crystallise or extract only that part and make it into a remedy. One example of this happened with *Digitalis* (foxglove). A remedy for heart conditions was made from this plant, but initially it caused some problems as the balance was incorrect. Following further research, *Digoxin* is used successfully as a remedy today and has helped many patients.

Alfred often spoke of his in-depth knowledge of *Echinacea* and of the terrific natural antibiotic properties of this plant. I was present once while a famous Dutch professor was interviewing him and I shall never forget Alfred's answer to one of his questions. When the professor asked Alfred how many medications he worked with, he replied that by his calculation there were roughly 360 but there was only one medicine which could be used to treat a large variety of illnesses. He then started to list all the benefits he had witnessed from this wonderful herb, *Echinaforce* (*Echinacea*), over the years. I can reinforce this statement because, throughout the years I have been in practice, *Echinaforce* has been of tremendous help and even saved my own life when I was desperately ill in Australia.

Vogel's life was totally absorbed in his great work. His energy rubbed off on me and even now, when I become tired, I recall how he used to soldier on to learn as much as he could about the healing power of plants. I would often find him experimenting with manure in order to produce the best organic blend he could, which, in turn, would produce the best herbs. If the manure was inferior, he would throw it away.

After I decided to work with Alfred in Teufen, one day he asked me to sign a legal document pledging that I would adhere to his principles and ensure that I prepared the remedies by meticulously following his recipes. I felt honoured to do so, having witnessed how carefully they had been developed, and I still strive to maintain the high standards and superior quality that were established by my mentor.

As our work progressed, Alfred began to travel around the world as part of his efforts to discover even more about nature and to look for solutions where science had failed. For example, he visited parts of the world where indigenous people maintained their traditional lifestyles in an attempt to find out why there was no cancer, multiple sclerosis or other such problems present there. I often travelled with him, along with his daughter Ruth, and I have wonderful memories of the journeys and friends we made.

I particularly recall trips we made to Holland to encourage the people in my home country to eat more sensibly. During the Second World War, the chronic shortage of food meant that Dutch people's diet was severely restricted. Interestingly, there was little evidence of colitis, diverticulitis or coeliac disease during this period, as the only foodstuffs freely available then were high in roughage. After the war ended, however, there was an explosion of such illnesses, as people began to eat anything they could get their hands on and, needless to say, these foods frequently contained limited nutrition. Thousands of people in Holland attended Vogel's lectures over the years, as this little Swiss man not only spoke a lot of sense but also educated people in how to lead a happier and healthier life.

If you ever visit Alfred Vogel's birthplace in the little village of Aesch in Switzerland, you will find a museum opened there in his honour which houses many of the artifacts he collected during the course of his travels around the world. He was unstoppable in his efforts to find out about growing plants and, while on the road, if we ever had cause to wonder where he had disappeared to, he could usually be found in the local markets – whether it be in Peru, Guatemala, the Amazon or whichever country we were in at the time. His energy for work was quite remarkable.

I clearly remember how delighted he was on his return from East Africa after finding out about the remarkable benefits of *Spilanthes*. He handed me a small leaf and asked me to eat it. Immediately a strong astringent action took place in my mouth. He asked, 'Do you see how important this plant is for people who have thrush in their mouth or the chronic skin disorder lichen planus?' *Spilanthes mauritiana* is a weed that grows profusely in Kenya and Uganda. It is a complete remedy that is totally safe for animals and humans alike but, for insects and fish, it acts as a strong poison. The flowers of the *Spilanthes* resemble chamomile in size and are used by the natives to alleviate toothache. The Zulus chew it as a treatment for mouth ulcers then rub it into their gums, which encourages this amazing sensation in the mouth. This feeling is so strong that you immediately know it will work. In Cameroon, it is used as a relief for snake bites and also sometimes for bladder and kidney problems. *Spilanthol* is the quickest-acting ingredient in this brilliant plant and, externally, it can be used for the most seemingly incurable skin disorders or fungi. It offers almost instant relief and has been of the greatest help to many people. He was an expert in finding out about such plants from remote areas of the world.

Another discovery I remember was a little orange bud, which resembled a little lantern. When he opened up his hand, he said, 'Look, the seeds inside this bud are like your heart – this gives us a sign that this is a wonderful heart remedy.' Yet again, another incredible product was developed from one of his finds.

Many years ago he returned from his travels to the Far East with a small *Ginkgo biloba* tree. As he was telling me all the benefits of *Ginkgo biloba* and showing me one of its leaves, he said, 'Look, it almost resembles your brain – isn't it wonderful that this is beneficial for treating problems in that area.' He planted that little tree in the garden beside his house and researched it extensively. It was not until he was totally satisfied with the results that he put it on the market. Today, we would not know how to manage without *Ginkgo biloba*, which has been of tremendous help to countless people, for example in the treatment of strokes, headaches and depression. As Vogel says in his marvellous book *The Nature Doctor*, it is the only plant remedy we know that is so beneficial for the brain, central nervous system and vascular system.

During his life and travels, he had the opportunity to talk to the most wonderful teachers and professors who were interested both in his views and his in-depth knowledge of herbal medicine. The famous practitioners who influenced him include Bircher-Benner, Dr William Pfeiffer, Dr Ragnar Berg and Dr Klopfer – all extremely knowledgeable people. I was lucky enough to meet some of them, too, and we had a most interesting time when we visited the Bircher-Benner, Willmar Schwabe and Joseph Issler clinics. As we watched the staff there at work, we were amazed to witness what could be done to alleviate human suffering.

Before he died, Vogel kindly passed on to me some books which are now a cherished part of my own collection. One of these was by Vogel himself – a wonderful volume called *The Tropical Guide of Nature Cure*. Sadly this book is no longer in print but it has been helpful to many people affected by seemingly incurable tropical diseases. During a visit to the Royal Tropical Institute in Amsterdam, I once witnessed a man suffering from bilharzia who was near to death; the remedies that Vogel prescribed to sort this man out and get the condition completely under control were remarkable.

Another of the books that Vogel passed on to me was the enormously influential environmental treatise *The Silent Spring* by Rachel Carson. Vogel took a great interest in what was happening around the world and was very concerned about environmental issues; climate change in particular caused him a lot of worry later in life. He was deeply influenced by what Rachel Carson had to say and he tried to share his concerns with as many people as possible. While in Australia, for example, we gave a talk on the dangers of DDT, which Carson had highlighted in her book as a dangerous pesticide that was having a detrimental effect on wildlife around the world. A group of young people came to speak to us afterwards and asked if there was anything they could do to help with this problem. I still remember Vogel encouraging them to tackle their government and to do all they could to try and get it banned. Eventually, due in large part to their campaign, Australia prohibited the use of DDT. Vogel spoke with such conviction that he inspired people to action.

Once, when we were in Biel-Bienne, he was asked to give two very important lectures. He prepared the gist of these in his mind, but when the organisers of the conference insisted that he wrote his lectures down, he was stuck! There would be people from 27 different nations attending that conference and so the translators obviously wanted a written lecture to work from; but as Vogel spoke from the heart, it was impossible for him to provide such a script. Although many lecturers require a lot of written material to prompt them, Vogel did his entirely off the cuff. His impromptu way of lecturing captivated his audiences and always received prolonged applause.

Vogel's greatest enemies were artificial manures, fertilisers, insecticides, pesticides and herbicides and I shall never forget the experiment he carried out which really taught us a lesson about the benefits of using natural versions of such products. He planted two cherry trees – one in a plot completely fed by organic means and which he took care of organically. The other tree was planted in a plot some distance from the first one, where it was encouraged to grow by the introduction of artificial insecticides and fed with artificial fertilisers – in fact, all the products Vogel disapproved of. A cherry tree does not usually have a long life, so, on one of my visits to Teufen, I was astounded to see that the tree he had planted in organic soil and fed organically was still alive and healthy. The other one had long since died. Also, while the artificially fed cherry tree had produced much larger cherries, they had no smell and little or no taste, whereas those from the organically cultivated tree were delicious. Again, he had shown that one has to cultivate plants naturally in order to create a good product; for Vogel, this was common sense and represented an investment in one's health.

In 1982, Alfred's devoted and faithful wife Sophie died. Together with their daughter Ruth, she and Alfred had spent their lives exploring nature and developing helpful remedies, and he was devastated by her death. I could see that he was really suffering, so I asked him to come to Scotland – as I knew he had enjoyed previous trips here – and my manageress, Janice Thompson, and my wife spent a great deal of time trying to console him. In an effort to distract his mind from his great loss, they took him to places like Culzean Castle, where he was shown many of the native plants of Scotland as well as some more exotic species from other countries.

Later, after some time had passed, Alfred was fortunate enough to meet Denise, who spent time trying to lift his spirits, until eventually happiness arose again and they were married. She too was very much in tune with his ideas, his faith and his hopes for the future. What the future held for them personally was joy. Denise also helped with the vast amount of correspondence and writing that he did in order to help other people.

Alfred made his last visit to Scotland in 1992. He thoroughly enjoyed walking in our gardens at Auchenkyle and was delighted when he saw the organic nursery we had established. We showed him the foods that were grown artificially for research, the foods that were grown organically and also the reports from the Scottish Agricultural College at Auchincruive detailing the high quality of vitamins, minerals and trace elements found in our organic produce. That made him very happy but he could not resist telling our gardeners how to prepare the soil and how to protect it from the extremely strong sunshine (he told them to cover it with straw to keep the bacteria in the ground, so that the produce from it would be of high quality). Then he turned his attention to the amount of money we were wasting in heating the glasshouses. His mind was still so alert that he said, 'If you dig down about four or five metres into the ground, you will probably find hot water and that will heat your glasshouses.' Of course, he turned out to be right and thanks to him we developed a very cheap method of heating. Alfred was a very practical man and was often able to advise us of possibilities that we had overlooked.

I once visited the Bioforce factory in Roggwil in Switzerland when they were making *Santasapina*, one of the most effective cough mixtures available, which is made from pine kernels. Vogel was a very thrifty man and could not bear to throw away the residue after the cough mixture had been made. He said, 'We can use these remains to extract aromatic oils which will be very beneficial for skin problems.' As far as Vogel was concerned, no natural product should ever be wasted.

On one occasion, I asked to have his IQ tested. I can't remember the exact score but I do recall that it was very high and that the professor who carried out the test told me, 'You are dealing with a genius.' That is exactly what he was and in the following chapters, I will explain a little bit more about the work we did together and the help we always tried to give to the countless people who were in need.

Chapter 2

Illness and suffering are caused by imbalance and disharmony, in whatever areas of our life they may occur.

Alfred Vogel

Alfred Vogel and I shared the view that it is vitally important in life to get the balance right. If we have a negative thought, then we must try and cancel this out with a positive thought. If there is an imbalance in one's health, then there are reasons for this and we must do everything possible to restore that balance. Just as an unbalanced wheel will cause a watch to stop, or an unbalanced load will cause a ship to capsize, so an imbalanced body will cause innumerable ailments in a human being. The centre of gravity of the body should always be in the correct position. The spine divides the body into left and right, and I often find it crucial to carry out spinal manipulation and spinal corrections to ensure the body is balanced.

In order to achieve balance for our patients, Vogel and I also agreed that, in many cases, they would benefit from a period during which they were under our constant care. In the late 1950s, Vogel had bought a lovely old house called Roode Wald in the beautiful rural setting of Nunspeet in Holland, right on the edge of the forest. I shared with him his vision of setting up the first nature cure clinic in the Netherlands and was delighted to join him in his work there. Roode Wald became a peaceful haven where many patients enjoyed the best care and attention. I have written about the clinic at length in the other volumes of my autobiography and I am still of the opinion that it was the finest place in which to look after people's well-being. As the patients were in our care for a set period of time, we were able to care for them holistically: combining a carefully monitored dietary regime with hands-on work such as massage and manipulation – and all treatments were purposely chosen to establish the balance between negative and positive.

I have often said that the future of medicine is in light and energy, and Vogel and I agreed that it was vital that the energy in all the rooms in the residential clinic was balanced. This became even clearer to us after we became familiar with the work of a gentleman called Nicolaas Kroeze. He was a well-known figure in Holland in his day, being the owner of a famous restaurant called The Five Flies. The Five Flies was widely acknowledged as being an outstanding and exclusive restaurant. It was wonderful to go there because every chair had a plaque on it giving the names of famous politicians, actors, film stars, sportspeople, etc. who had sat there. It had a great atmosphere and I can remember Vogel and I spending a most enjoyable evening there.

Nicolaas Kroeze came to Roode Wald to have a look around shortly after we opened. He had very specific ideas about negative and positive energy, and told us that, completely unaided, he had built a special glasshouse in his garden. He had thoroughly checked the energy lines under the glasshouse so that everything from the foundation upwards was in balance. After completing his construction, he saw his first patient there – a 12-year-old girl with leukaemia who, he told us, had been totally cured by the sun's rays and by the well-balanced energy that existed in that glasshouse. I am sure, as was Vogel, that Nicolaas Kroeze was another man who was ahead of his time. It was disappointing that he never got the backing to continue his work and substantiate his claims, and I still feel there is enormous scope for research into the work that he started.

This story made us realise that we should examine several rooms and areas in our clinic where we thought that the energy might be out of balance. We contacted another pioneering gentleman who arrived with apparatus that he had invented himself which could measure the energy forces in each room. He came to the conclusion that, apart from one room, the clinic was actually well balanced. The problematic space was a small room in which, he said, a faulty energy line from the earth went straight through the bed. He therefore advised us that it would be wiser to either change the position of the bed or not to use the room at all. We had, in fact, already noticed that people who used that room did not respond so well to treatment and we had made the decision not to use that room for consultations but merely for storage – that, incidentally, was entirely through our own intuition. This was a most interesting exercise and, as I have said, we had outstanding successes in that clinic.

When a geologist carried out a similar test in my own clinic, Mokoia, which I opened in Troon in 1970, he also found that there were two places where, as he put it, the 'holy energy lines were not in balance'. I refused to use these rooms to treat patients and I remain convinced that energy is the future of medicine.

Another pioneering step we took at Roode Wald involved colonic irrigation. This was a popular treatment back in the 1960s and has enjoyed a recent resurgence. An eminent Dutch professor, who had heard about our work, stepped into our clinic one day. After having a look around, he remarked how impressed he was and told us that he was keen to demonstrate his views on how to clear the 'inner chemistry' of the body. He asked if he could undertake some research work in our premises and when we pressed him for further details, he said he wanted to set up some apparatus to facilitate what he called 'higher bowel cleansing'. He told us that a rigorous detoxification programme would require the body to be thoroughly cleaned out.

We agreed to his proposal and so, for a short time, he worked with us on a voluntary basis to demonstrate the long-established principles of colonic irrigation, practised in his own, very thorough, way. He was busy for many weeks setting things up and, finally, when he was ready to start consulting, he showed us his fairly monstrous-looking apparatus and the procedure involved. Although this was something new to us, we trusted him because he was a professor of medicine.

His first patient was an extremely overweight lady. The

process entailed having about 40 pints of chamomile water flushed through her system in order to totally cleanse her bowel. When he had finished, he showed us almost half a bucket of waste material that had been flushed out of her bowel and explained that the retention of such waste was a major cause of ill heath. Too much waste material in the bowel can encourage the excessive growth of a yeast or fungus, either of which definitely makes people ill. It is essential that the bowels are clean and that people have a motion every day. What you import in 24 hours, you have to export in 24 hours or even sooner; otherwise you are inviting problems. Our inner chemistry is most important.

The professor did the most wonderful job at the clinic, staying with us for about a year, and he told us that, just as people give their homes a thorough clean in spring and autumn, they should do likewise with their 'house of health'. This, he told us, would be extremely beneficial in helping to maintain health and harmony in the body. My own grandmother had also always stressed the importance of regular bowel movements and advised people when they had problems with their bowels, or even the slightest constipation, to take castor oil.

When I asked Vogel for his views on colonic irrigation, he said it was probably all right to carry it out every now and then but the danger was that people could become addicted, as they felt so well and energetic after it. In fact, he had a patient who wanted to carry out the procedure every day. This can have a detrimental effect on the function of the intestine, as it will flush out the healthy bacteria along with any waste matter. The intestine must be given time to recover after each treatment. If we eat a well-balanced diet and there is perhaps only a slight problem with constipation, then there are some excellent simple remedies, such as *Linoforce*, that can be taken to clean out the system.

Colonic irrigation was helpful for people who were grossly overweight and another successful method that we introduced to help weight control was our fasting days. Vogel was very keen on fasting but he always said that one had to do it sensibly. For those patients who stayed in the clinic, one day per week was a fasting, or juice, day. Interestingly, when people followed this regime – which involved having a glass of either vegetable or fruit juice for breakfast, lunch, dinner and supper – they felt so much better the following day. Everything in life needs balance, and balancing the human body is one of the most beneficial things to do to promote good health. Fasting allows the body to rebalance itself through detoxification.

Although the clinic in Nunspeet was a thriving business, it was by no means easy to manage. Vogel and I worked day and night to provide the necessary care but we struggled to employ qualified back-up staff to assist us. Finding other practitioners who were equally devoted to alleviating human suffering was much more difficult than we had expected. We encountered doctors who were unreliable and nurses who were often too busy with other things to do their job properly. We had no end of problems with domestic and kitchen staff, and some people stole from us – I could go on and on.

Vogel and I frequently held meetings to see if we could figure out how to improve the running of the business and I remember one such meeting that went on until nearly one o'clock in the morning. Vogel always rose very early –

sometimes as early as four or five o'clock – and he always liked to go to bed between nine and ten o'clock at night or even earlier. He had an extremely long working day and that particular night I could see that he was beginning to get tired. Even though all the staff members had had ample opportunity to express their thoughts on the matter at hand, there was still no resolution in sight. Finally, he said, 'Let's reach a united decision. Let "yes" mean "yes" and "no" mean "no".' In other words, he wanted them to be decisive. He wanted things to be set out in black and white. They should consider their individual responsibilities and decide on the best course of action; then they should be resolute in their decision. Vogel had no time for indecision and never used half-hearted measures when tackling problems but dealt with them head on. Life would be much more straightforward if everyone stuck to the principle whereby 'yes' means 'yes' and 'no' means 'no'. Unfortunately, in today's society there appear to be so many grey areas and people often lack the backbone to stand up for their decisions.

As well as problems with staff, we also encountered resistance from the governmental authorities about the work we were doing in the clinic and in August 1961 I was summoned, along with three of the doctors who were working in the clinic at the time, to a meeting with the Dutch Inspector of Health in Nijmegen. At the meeting, the three of us who were able to attend were told in no uncertain terms that we should not continue with our work. The medical establishment was completely opposed to natural medicine and any clinics that did not follow the orthodox methods of treatment. The official threatened to take away our licences to practise and warned that if we refused to comply, we could face imprisonment. It appeared to be the government's intention to shut down the clinic.

When I told Vogel about our encounter with this bureaucrat, he encouraged me to stand firm and said, 'Good will always triumph in the end.' Unfortunately, however, my colleagues in the clinic decided to give up. They were too frightened to ignore the threats, as they did not want to risk losing their licences. For men with young families to support, this was an understandable decision but I myself resolved to keep going. This was not an easy decision to make and there continued to be a lot of governmental interference and threats. We incurred a lot of unnecessary expense due to these problems and, added to the terrific staffing problems that we were already experiencing, it became very difficult to carry on.

Eventually, as a result of all these problems, we were forced to change the clinic into one for day care only. I was determined, however, that whatever difficulties we were facing, the medicines developed by Vogel over so many years would not be allowed to disappear or be forced off the Dutch market and fought very hard for their continued existence. Thankfully, many of those medicines are nowadays being prescribed by a high percentage of doctors in Holland and are even being administered in hospitals. It was a tremendous achievement to win that fight.

Another product which survived was the famous 'Vogel bread'. This was an important part of the balanced diet which Vogel recommended to patients at the clinic. The bread was made from his own recipe, baked from whole grains, not crushed, and was absolutely delicious. This bread was already popular before a chance conversation in the clinic one day led to it being improved.

Our visitor on this occasion was the owner of a large bakery in Holland called Het Zeeuwse Meisje. Vogel asked me a few questions during this meeting and I joined in the conversation by telling both men a story about my youth. I must have been about six or seven years old, as the Second World War was still raging through Europe and Holland was occupied by the Nazis. There was very little to eat during the war years and one day my constant hunger got me into trouble. While I was out in the street, I saw a Nazi soldier eating some bread and watched as he threw the crust onto the street. My mother had told me very strictly never to take anything from the Nazis, or from the Dutch collaborators, but I was so hungry that I snatched that discarded crust of bread from the gutter and devoured it. I thought it was the best thing I had ever tasted. It had a particularly sour flavour but I was too young then to analyse what was in it. Nevertheless, it was delicious. When I arrived back home, I owned up to my mother what I had done and was punished severely.

As I told both men this story, the baker's eyes suddenly lit up and he said, 'I know what the Germans put into that bread during the war to make their soldiers healthy and strong – that was a very good recipe.' Vogel was so pleased to hear this story because he understood exactly what the baker was speaking about: the secret ingredient was whole rye. They both investigated this thoroughly and, as a result, Vogel adapted his bread-making recipe to make it even more beneficial for health.

Vogel's bread is still available today, providing an important part of a balanced diet, and it is with the greatest of pleasure that I can report that Dr Vogel's cereals are also available in Britain. These formulas have been brilliantly put together by a company called Britannia Health and it is wonderful to see this nutritious, delicious and gluten-free cereal, which is of particular benefit to patients suffering with multiple sclerosis and coeliac disease, on the British market.

Grabbing a quick, nutritious bowl of cereal before rushing out of the house in the morning is the normal way to kick-start the day for much of the population. But this is not an option for an estimated 250,000 people in the UK with coeliac disease who are unable to tolerate the wheat, barley, rye and oats found in most cereals.

New VitaPro is a great-tasting, 'stay crunchy' alternative for coeliacs and others with gluten intolerance. VitaPro is a vitamin- and protein-enriched soy cereal, flavoured with natural honey and cinnamon. It is also the first breakfast cereal in the UK to contain Hi-maize, a unique and completely natural functional food ingredient rich in resistant starch, fibre and probiotic properties which significantly improve bowel health. Other fantastic products are Soytana and Ultrabran.

Alfred and I did some wonderful work at Roode Wald and we had great opportunities there to experiment and meet people from very varied backgrounds who shared with us some brilliant ideas. It was such a pity that the clinic was only open for a short time. We strived to help our patients achieve a healthy balance in their lives and were determined to carry on providing people with advice through our lectures and books. It is sometimes difficult for people to find the help they are looking for and that is why I have now written over 40 books dealing with many different issues. It is also wonderful to be able to back up this advice with the helpful remedies that Vogel devised and such products as his bread and cereals.

Chapter 3

Happiness is the soothing balm for a sick heart
and the best remedy for a wounded heart.

Alfred Vogel

It is now almost 45 years since Vogel and I first discussed in detail the subject of happiness and the importance of maintaining a positive mental attitude. While working in the clinic at Roode Wald one day in May 1961, I received a phone call from Switzerland to say that Vogel was urgently needed, as they were making an important decision there that required his input. He had gone to Amsterdam unexpectedly, so I was not sure exactly where to find him, but it was obviously vital that I did so.

After many fruitless enquiries, I eventually managed to track him down to the home of a very unhappy couple whose daughter had been told that she only had a few months to live. He had gone to offer them help and comfort, and was doing all he could for these people in their time of need. On my arrival,

I relayed the message that he had to phone Switzerland immediately and so we had to leave. But even during the short time that I was there I could see that the family had derived reassurance and comfort from Vogel's personal visit. Fortunately, it would also transpire that the remedies Vogel prescribed had a beneficial effect on the daughter's immune system.

He felt extremely relieved that he had managed to help them but on the return journey to the clinic at Nunspeet he discussed the huge impact that the daughter's illness had had on the whole family. He explained to me that these people were worried to death about their daughter. We discussed the meaning of this phrase and Alfred explained that there are circumstances in life where worrying can spiral out of control. When this happens, it can have a serious effect on a person's health, causing stress which can lead to heart attacks, high blood pressure, strokes and so on. In severe cases, people can literally worry themselves to death. With the family we had just visited, not only were they dealing with the daughter's illness but also the effects of the intense stress that they were all under – and in some cases, worrying about an illness can actually cause more harm than the illness itself.

I wholeheartedly agreed that constant worry not only physically affects the body but also eats away at the soul of Man. In such instances, it is vital that people find some way to be positive about the circumstances in which they find themselves, however difficult this may appear to be. This is a vital part of achieving the balance that I discussed in the previous chapter.

I always admired the way in which Vogel coped with great

problems by trying to remain positive and maintaining that glimmer of happiness which helped him through life's journeys. The quote at the beginning of this chapter has remained at the forefront of my mind over the years and he also told me that that happiness will be inexhaustible once you have found it.

There are many things in life that can make one *un*happy – selfishness, resentment, jealousy, envy, unhappy marriages, work and stress, for example. How often do I hear people moaning, 'Oh no, yet another day – I will need to try and get through it,' or 'Work again – I would rather be on holiday,' or 'I only look forward to the weekend.' There are many people who wake up with such feelings of dread and then turn over and try to go back to sleep for as long as possible. People like this are wishing their lives away.

I see the results of such negative attitudes every day in my clinics and I treat increasing numbers of patients for problems associated with their nervous systems. This is a sign that something in their body is not functioning properly but it is also often related to their outlook on life. If one makes an effort to go to bed at a reasonable time and waken up in the morning feeling and acting positively, then one can go to work in a happy frame of mind. It is also important to combine such a positive attitude with a healthy breakfast. If nerves are beginning to affect your life, then I would suggest having porridge for breakfast, together with plenty of fruit and vegetables, which will give the system a terrific boost to start the day. Only by being optimistic each day, working to the best of one's ability and finding satisfaction at the end of it can one experience real joy.

The other day I saw a recovered cancer patient. He looked at me and said, 'You know, I am grateful now for every day that God gives me, for the simple reason that I have been given an extension to my life and I am going to make the best of it.' That is really the most important thing anyone can do.

Each day should be seen as a gift and if we continue to be pessimistic, we encourage some extremely nasty diseases to develop. For example, I am convinced through research I have undertaken that cancer is influenced by the mind, both positively and negatively. Through visualisation techniques, meditation and positive thinking, a cancer patient can survive longer or, more amazingly, beat cancer entirely. The reverse side to this is that a negative attitude may well exacerbate the problem.

Back in 1961, during the journey from Amsterdam with Vogel, he described the physical effects that a positive state of mind can have on the body: for example, the pancreas will begin to function more effectively; the secretion of digestive enzymes increases, allowing the body to absorb nutrition from food more effectively; and, above all, it can improve liver function, as the liver is very sensitive to any emotional imbalance. Even if you feel unhappy, you should breathe in and out with the mental awareness that happiness is like warmth and can warm even the coldest heart. Happiness brings us peace, it improves attitudes and is a soothing balm that helps us to combat health problems. Happiness is also beneficial for the circulatory system. The sympathetic nervous system and all the organs that are related to it will gladly do their job if one is relaxed and happy. My grandmother always used to say that a patient will only get better if he is in a state of relaxation.

Following a virus I contracted while in the bush in Australia, which affected my pancreas, I sadly developed diabetes. It is vital that diabetics have a positive outlook and keep their spirits up, and one genuine comfort I have is that I am able to control my diabetes without the use of any insulin or other drugs. This is thanks to the natural remedies that I use and the healthy, positive way I try to lead my life. I feel very thankful for this wonderful creation in which we live – where every plant, every flower and every tree bark can tell us a story and often offer a solution to a problem. Although that viral enemy in the bush tried to destroy the contentment within me, I managed to overcome that force with the countless positive thoughts that I have put into my life and this buoyant attitude has also enabled me to continue to work 90 hours a week and remain happy.

One problem with a heavy workload of this kind is that it means that sacrifices have to be made in some other areas of life. Alfred Vogel dedicated himself totally to his work and helping other people. I can understand why he worked so tirelessly and have followed the same path myself. However, by devoting myself to helping others, this has meant that I have been unable to spend as much time as I would have liked at home with my wife and my children. Sometimes when I reflect on this reality it makes me very unhappy, but then there is often some light to follow such dark thoughts.

The other day, for example, I received a little thank you card from one of my daughters, which said, 'We want to thank you, not only for the hard work that you have done all your life to help others, but also in helping us, because we would not be where we are today if it hadn't been for your hard work.' Such thoughtful gestures make all the toil and sacrifice feel worthwhile and enable me to keep moving on, looking forward to everything that life still holds in store for me.

I remember when Vogel came over after my second daughter was born. He held her in his arms and, beaming with pleasure, said, 'Isn't creation wonderful? Look at the perfection of this newborn child. Perhaps one day, she will work with us to make a lot of people happy.' That same child is now the managing director of one of our companies, Bioforce UK.

There are so many healing powers all around us and such a lot that we can do to help ourselves achieve better health by embracing happiness in our lives. Gloria Hunniford, who I worked with on many occasions, gave me some good advice when we were facing some difficulties. She told me, 'My dear mother always said, "If you have problems or worries, tackle them positively. If you cannot sort them out, leave them alone and they will sort themselves out."' Life's problems can often be resolved by adopting this kind of positive attitude and another thing that can help is having a good sense of humour.

When I arrived in Scotland in 1970, being Dutch I knew nothing about the dry Scottish sense of humour. Over the years, however, I have come to understand that style of humour and am now of the opinion that it is probably the best in the world. Often during the days when I am in practice in my clinics in Scotland I can be cheered up by the witty comments that patients make.

Vogel also had a great sense of humour, which came as a surprise to me because, like the Dutch, the Swiss are not renowned for their wit! Possibly it is because both nationalities are too conscientious. While this is a very good quality, if we lose our sense of humour, we miss out on an awful lot in life.

In the evening, as we ponder the day's events, the parts that stick in our mind are probably those joyful instances that have helped improve our day and made us laugh. On the other hand, some people go a little bit too far in the other direction, by trying to laugh off any problems with forced humour. Laughter is a wonderful thing but it should come naturally and not be forced.

In 1961, when Vogel and I were first discussing the importance of happiness and positivity, Seasonal Affective Disorder (SAD) was unheard of. Today, however, it is becoming a serious issue with an estimated half a million people in the UK suffering from this type of depression every winter. SAD is caused by a biochemical imbalance in the hypothalamus, which in turn is caused by the reduced hours of daylight and lack of sunshine we have here in Britain, particularly between December and February. While I have a great deal of sympathy for people suffering from this condition, I often wonder whether part of the problem is that they have lost the ability to find simple pleasure in looking around at this great creation.

It is often the little things in life that make one happy. I frequently think of my own grandmother, who was equally wise as Dr Vogel and equally happy. She often advised that when a problem or some unhappiness arose, then one should look out of the window at this great creation of which we are all part and, even at the gloomiest of moments, to try and sing a song.

We must always remember that sun is still there behind all the dark clouds. I advise people, if at all possible, to try to save up for a conservatory and expose themselves to as much light as possible. This exposure – particularly to natural daylight around midday – can be of great benefit to those suffering from winter depression.

Light is a very important part of life and while thinking about how to maintain happiness and defeat depression, I frequently turn to a biblical expression that I have discussed in many of my previous books: once we have found the light on our pathway, if we walk in that light, we will become children of the light. I once discussed this with an eminent scientist, Professor Arthur Ellison, who said that he believed that light and energy would be significant in the future of medicine. We need to energise ourselves and be aware of the ways in which we can improve our way of life. This will enable us to attain a much deeper, more satisfying joy, which will help us as we carry out our daily duties.

When I was only 18, more than 50 years ago, I was fortunate enough to assist a renowned professor in a local hospital. The matron who worked there always appeared to be happy and smiling. She kept the whole place running like clockwork, and, unlike modern hospitals in the UK, there were never any problems connected to hygiene because she ensured the wards were spotless. She used to paraphrase an old biblical expression, saying, 'Be careful, because unhappiness is a rotting of bones.' There was a wonderful atmosphere in that hospital because even though this matron had an extremely responsible and stressful job she still displayed such a happy attitude that it rubbed off on the staff and others around her. It is encouraging to see that, when we are happy, we touch the hearts of others and then this happiness, in turn, is passed on.

Back on that journey from Amsterdam all those years ago,

Vogel explained how negative influences such as ignorance, inexperience, bad attitudes, neglect and evil thoughts can dampen our enthusiasm for life and lead to sadness and depression. He stressed how important it is that we continue to be optimistic, and quoted an old saying: 'The happiness we give to others will return to make our own hearts rejoice.'

Happiness for Vogel that day had been achieved by making the effort to find that simple little house in the middle of Amsterdam and helping to relieve the family of some of their burden of sorrow. It was instances like that that Vogel found so fulfilling and, no matter where he was, he would do whatever he could to bring happiness to others.

Chapter 4

This is really the essence of life – by trying to help others, we, in turn, help ourselves.

Alfred Vogel

While emphasising the importance of being happy and maintaining a positive attitude, it is also necessary to recognise that sometimes events in life overtake us and even the most positive people can succumb to the effects of depression. Some of the most enlightening conversations about this problem and the ways to overcome it took place between two of my best friends, Jos Lussenburg and Alfred Vogel.

Jos and I became great friends when we lived in Nunspeet. My whole family adored him and while my children were growing up, he was like a grandfather to them. He would come to visit me every morning on his bicycle and we would have long talks. We had a special bond of friendship that helped both of us in dealing with our respective problems in life. I therefore understood him very well and when he mentioned his interest in talking to Alfred Vogel, I was very happy to set up a meeting between these two great thinkers one beautiful summer evening. They hit it off very well and were able to talk freely to one another. I felt privileged to be there and was greatly encouraged by many of the different things that they said.

Jos was a very talented artist and musician, and he was a pillar of the community, carrying out a lot of charitable work in the small town where we lived. But behind Jos's wonderful warm face, not everything in his life was rosy.

Jos had harnessed his musical talent and worked hard at his craft to become a famous professional violinist. When he was at the height of his music career, however, he lost two of his fingertips as the result of an infection. This did not diminish the love that he had for music, and indeed he was still able to play and conduct, but the fact that his ability had been impaired devastated him to such an extent that he became deeply depressed.

Today, when I see portraits of Beethoven, I can understand how artists struggled to capture the expressions on that great composer's face, as he was equally depressed when he lost his hearing. Like Beethoven, music was Lussenburg's great passion and, possibly as a result of his disability, he was able to express more powerful emotions when playing his violin or piano than many able-bodied musicians were capable of.

After the accident, not even aware that he could draw, Jos decided to take up painting. As he developed his skills, he began to realise that that although one can put one's thoughts into one's music, one can express oneself even more deeply in painting. Jos became an extremely successful artist, with his paintings being sold for tremendous sums of money.

That evening, as he spoke to Alfred Vogel about his health and the several depressive periods that had darkened his life, it was fascinating to hear Vogel tell Jos that he had met several famous artists – using the term to cover those gifted in music, painting, singing, etc. – during his career and they all had one thing in common: because of their exceptional gift, they sometimes suffered from bouts of deep depression.

Fortunately, though, Lussenburg was not the type of man to stay depressed for long and while at times his talents could lead him to frustration and desolation, at other points they brought him great joy and comfort. He told Vogel that, whether painting or just sitting by the riverbank, he experienced a terrific release from life's tensions when he thought of Beethoven and all that he achieved. He proudly claimed to have all his symphonies, but felt that the 5th was a particularly wonderful piece and declared that he knew the 7th off by heart.

On that warm summer evening, when the three of us were in Lussenburg's home, we talked together about the disharmonies in life and how music and, for Lussenburg, also his paintings, managed to bring it all back into balance. Lussenburg often said to me that depression is a state of mind and you need to muster up as much strength as possible to overcome it. We agreed that one's outlook can be positively changed by the therapeutic influence of music, even by singing a song when depression surfaces. Although they both suffered from this affliction, Mozart's and Beethoven's wonderful melodies have helped countless others overcome depression. It is important, though, to choose the right type of music to deal with each individual situation. The tranquillity of a soft melody can make the stormiest heart calm and possibly happy again.

Jos also enjoyed going sailing and he told us that when he went out on his boat, he sang a song that went, 'When my ship went out of the harbour, roll on my ship, roll on my ship, back to the home haven again'. His house was actually called '*Thuishaven*' (which literally means 'home haven'). As Lussenburg grew up next to the sea, he understood it very well and could paint seascapes like no one else. Vogel was very interested in this story, and as they were talking about life's problems and whether one could find peace in music or in painting, Lussenburg gave one of his paintings to Vogel.

That night they talked about the significance of life and how important it was for everyone to be grateful to the Creator. As Lussenburg said, 'God rules the traffic and it is important that, as we all move around, we remember that the great captain will determine the course of our lives.' In this great universe where we can be compared to a small drop in the ocean, we should realise that we are still part of that ocean and belong to it. Perhaps we are all guilty of not fully appreciating gifts that we receive. We should be thankful every day for those wonderful gifts of light, sunshine, air and nature that so many of us take for granted.

We all agreed that one has to be realistic by facing the problems we encounter along the way and making the best of them. Life is a miracle, and if we accept it as such, then we will be able to embark upon each day as a new challenge. Even when in his 90s, that is what Vogel did, and Lussenburg too, when he was in his 80s.

'How can an ill person be happy?' was one of the questions that was discussed that summer evening. It is often remarkable to see how some people, once they have come to terms with their illness, can be such a positive example to others and can spread much happiness to those around them. I have personally seen many critically ill people who, although accepting that they were coming to the end of their lives, still endeavoured to maintain a positive attitude and it is comforting to think that such people, no matter how little they have left to give, can still be such a help to others. To have a desire to help others is a commendable attitude.

My mother used to say, 'If you look around, you will always find somebody who is worse off than you.' I feel great sympathy in my heart when I see people struggling with their health problems – particularly those with degenerative diseases such as cancer, multiple sclerosis, muscular dystrophy or those crippled by osteoarthritis or rheumatoid arthritis. Although life can be particularly miserable for many such people, moaning and groaning about it cannot change things, whereas having a happy attitude will not only help oneself, but also those around us.

When one exerts oneself to find inner harmony in the three bodies that Man has, then one is equipped to find unending happiness. It makes such a difference when we open our windows in the morning with a happy heart. We should realise that we are all part of this great creation and see each day ahead as a challenge.

When my two friends talked about their trips around the world, Vogel told Lussenburg all about his great experiences in Peru. While there, he observed some of the world's poorest people but, surprisingly, they still appeared to be happy. When they suffered from illnesses and diseases, they took it into their own hands to regain their health, harnessing the power of the wonderful natural ingredients around them. When he went to the herbal markets in Peru and saw the huge variety of herbs being sold there, Vogel realised that the power for healing that God had provided through nature made these people happy and appreciative of the little they had. Their gratitude was written on their faces and, when Vogel went amongst them to offer advice, it made him happy that he was able to assist these underprivileged people. As he said, 'This is really the essence of life – by trying to help others, we, in turn, help ourselves.' The simple saying, 'you get out of life what you put into it' is also, in most cases, so true.

We talked that evening about some wonderful remedies that Vogel found throughout the world – not only in Peru but in many other countries – and the relief that such treatment could have on balancing nervous anxieties and depression. Of course, Vogel and Lussenburg thought highly of the plant *St John's Wort* for its characteristics and signatures. This herb, named after the apostle of love, St John, has lifted the spirits of many people. Even Paracelsus recognised that it was a mood enhancer. What a wonderful gift this plant has been. If we take one of its leaves and study it under a microscope, we can see it is filled with a wonderful substance called *St John's Wort* oil. Today, however, *St John's Wort* is seen as a great threat to the powerful tranquillisers and antidepressants produced by the drugs industry and has, astonishingly, been banned in some countries.

When we went out into Lussenburg's peaceful garden, Vogel pointed out such plants as the sweet chestnut, clematis, rock rose, honeysuckle and gentian, the oak and the elm, all flowering and growing profusely – and he told us of the tremendous healing powers of those plants, flowers, herbs and trees. They are a valuable part of creation and, by their signatures and characteristics, they show us what they should be used for. I was able to harness the power of many flowers in my range of flower essences. These are liquid extracts of flowers in a base of grape alcohol. They can be taken orally and can have a beneficial effect on the emotions – which, in turn, can be beneficial for the health of the whole body.

While listening to Alfred and Jos in the surroundings of Lussenburg's studio, I counted myself blessed to be in their company. They were both recalling memorable occasions and were thankful that they had been given the opportunity to experience so much during their busy lives. Both had many interests and so much to do in their work that they never became bored, and the inheritance they left behind and their wonderful spirits are still with us today, helping many people.

I really like the word 'enthusiasm'. In one dictionary I have, it gives its meaning as 'God in you' – and this enthusiasm was clearly evident in those two special gentlemen that evening. Enthusiasm for helping others in today's world is very important, as is recognising that God can work within us in this great creation to bring happiness and good health into all our lives. That was the important lesson I learned that evening, and I shall treasure it to the end of my days.

Chapter 5

Foresight is the source of health and happiness.
Alfred Vogel, 1902–96

At the time I graduated in the late 1950s, there were revolutionary changes going on in the pharmaceutical industry. The world was witnessing an explosion in the production of drugs such as antibiotics, tranquillisers and steroids, and these were being seized upon by the medical profession as some kind of panacea or holy grail. We were told that this was progress and that there would soon be a drug to treat every kind of ailment. While most people were very enthusiastic about these developments, I had serious reservations about the road the medical profession was travelling along. As far as I could see, these new drugs were created to treat specific symptoms that patients presented but little attempt seemed to be being made to establish why those problems had occurred in the first place. I worried that the widespread administration of such drugs would mean that major health problems in patients would merely be suppressed rather than addressed successfully. I foresaw a situation by which we would create chronic invalids who were dependent on synthetic drugs and I believe that today, with the spread of diseases such as ME and cancer, my predictions have been proved correct.

For obvious reasons, having such foresight often brings more frustration than satisfaction. It can be very difficult to get others to listen to your advice and you can feel helpless as you watch the problems that you have foreseen proliferate.

Vogel was a man with great foresight. When I look back to the work that he did when we opened the clinic at Nunspeet, I am always amazed at the way he was able to identify disorders that at that time were practically unheard of. He investigated problems that could arise in the body's yeast processes, such as the excessive growth of candida albicans, and he also conducted research into the pathogen helicobacter pylori, which can cause intestinal problems such as ulcers.

One of the most effective remedies Vogel created for sufferers of candida albicans and other yeast infections was developed from *Spilanthes*, one of his African discoveries which I have described previously. He would prescribe this along with a strict dietary regime. The juices had to be prepared from fresh vegetables and fruits using a juicer, and everything that was to be eaten had to be chewed thoroughly, so that it would mix properly with the saliva in one's mouth – a vital part of the digestive process. After following this regime, patients could slowly return to a more varied, natural diet. The programme he set up was very simple but very effective and I have detailed it below:

The first two days started with: Chamomile tea at 8 a.m.; freshly prepared fruit juice at 10 a.m.; vegetable juice at noon; Chamomile tea at 4 p.m.; and, at 6 p.m., fruit juice.

The following two days were made up of: Chamomile tea at 8 a.m.; yogurt at 10 a.m., together with some separate fruit juice; quark (soft white cheese) at noon; Chamomile tea again at 4 p.m.; and, at 6 p.m., quark with some separate fruit juice.

The next two to three days were: Chamomile tea and some Ryvita at 8 a.m.; fruit juice at 10 a.m.; buttermilk with some separate vegetable juice at noon; Chamomile tea and two pieces of Ryvita spread with a little butter at 4 p.m.; and, at 6 p.m., some muesli.

The next two to three days consisted of: Chamomile tea with two or three pieces of Ryvita at 8 a.m.; fruit juice with some separate quark at 10 a.m.; fruit juice and yogurt at noon; Chamomile tea with two slices of Ryvita at 4 p.m.; and, at 6 p.m., some muesli.

To be taken the next two to three days was: Chamomile tea with two Ryvitas spread with a little butter at 8 a.m.; muesli at 10 a.m.; raw vegetables with some boiled rice at noon; fruit juice and an egg at 4 p.m.; and, at 6 p.m., muesli with some Ryvita.

The subsequent two to three days were: Chamomile tea at 8 a.m. with Ryvita spread with a small amount of butter; muesli at 10 a.m.; raw vegetables with some boiled rice at noon; Chamomile tea plus two or three slices of Ryvita spread with a little butter; and, at 6 p.m., muesli and Ryvita.

I understand that people who followed this diet enjoyed relief from their symptoms and rarely suffered from any further problems with candida albicans or yeast-processing difficulties. While I have now identified other ways to treat candida albicans and helicobacter pylori, which are less restricting for patients, it is nevertheless fascinating to see how far advanced Vogel was all those years ago in dealing with uncommon problems that have become so widespread today.

I have taken this opportunity to include in the following pages some further examples of the balanced diets devised by Vogel for patients at Roode Wald.

I apologise for the fact that these diets are still in Dutch and German, but I wanted to show a snippet of his work to demonstrate how much effort was spent in putting those diets together.

Such strict dietary programmes highlight the importance which Vogel attached to nutritional advice – an area in which he was, once again, ahead of his time. As a pupil of Bircher-Benner, Vogel focused on creating a balanced diet for his patients and so everything that was done in the kitchens at his clinics came under his close scrutiny. I often heard him becoming extremely annoyed when the dieticians hadn't done something properly. He examined every diet personally to ensure that the carbohydrates and proteins were perfectly balanced and that the acid/alkaline balance was also in order. He was particularly concerned that all foods be organically grown and naturally produced.

He achieved great successes with this approach but it wasn't always easy to persuade people to follow his methods. I can still hear him saying, 'People can change their political party,

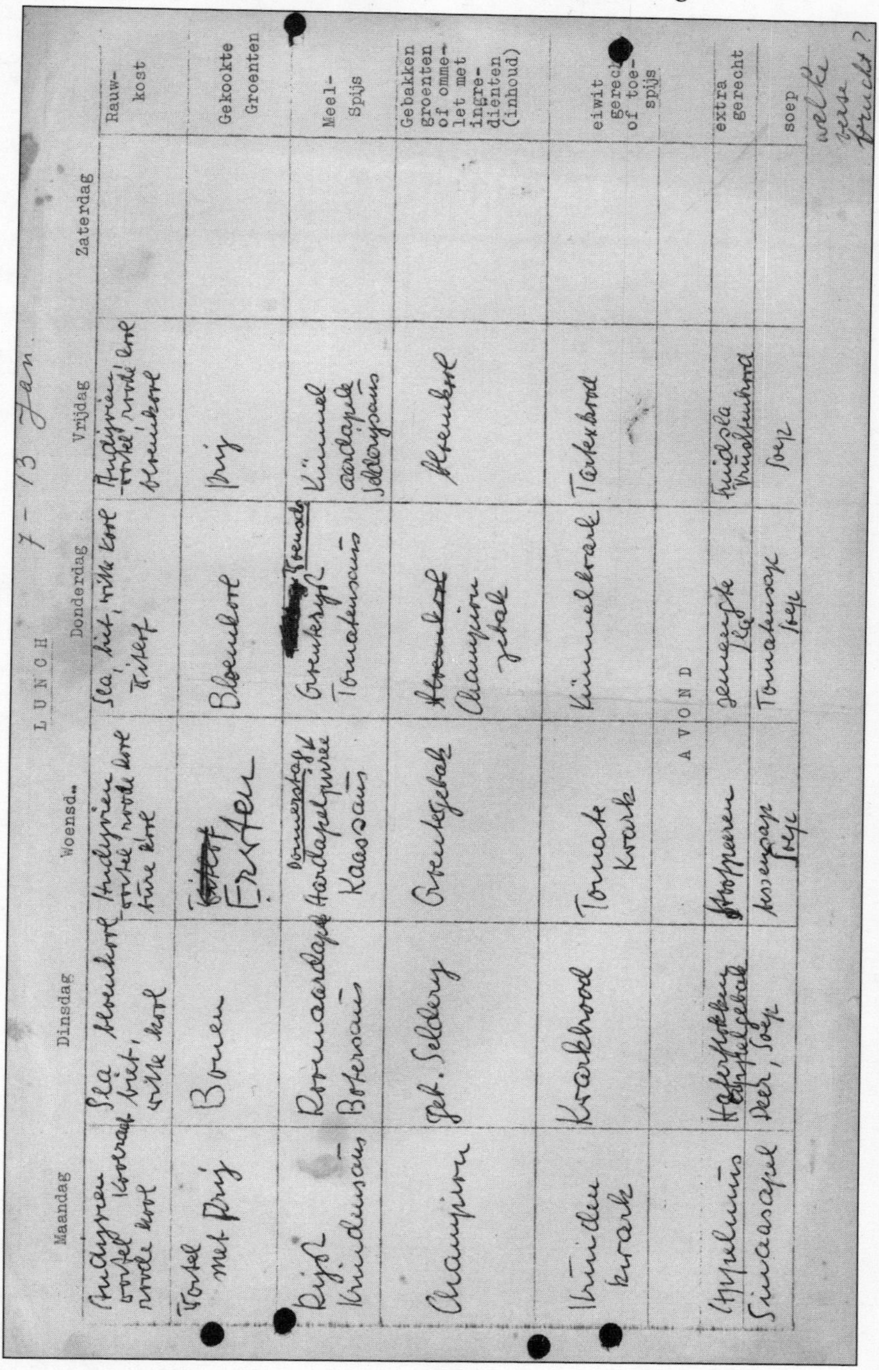

LUNCH   7 - 13 Jan.

	Maandag	Dinsdag	Woensd..	Donderdag	Vrijdag	Zaterdag	
Rauw-kost	Andijvie, witlof, wortel, witte kool	Sla, bleuselie, witlof, witte kool	Andijvie, witlof, witte kool, rauwe biet	Sla, biet, witte kool, zilverui	Andijvie, witlof, witte kool, bieulbeet		
Gekookte Groenten	Tortel met Prij	Boven	Stoof Eraten	Bloemkool	Prij		
Meel-Spijs	Rijst vruchensaus	Rauwaardap.- Botersaus	Bruine aardap, Hartappelpuree Kaassaus	Groenkryst Tomatensaus	Kümmel aardapel Seldrosaus		
Gebakken groenten of ommelet met ingredienten (inhoud)	Champion	gek. Seldery	Groentegehal	Stoomslat Champion gehal	Bloemkool		
eiwit gerecht of toe- spijs	Krielen Krack	Krackbrood	Tomaat Krack	Kümmelkrack	Tarkerbrod		
AVOND							
extra gerecht	Apulius Suicaracpul	Haferflokken Hafulgehol veel, Sap	Stroopeeren kassengap Joye	jeneverpr. Pr. Tomatensap joye	Frückcla Vruchtenbrod Sap		
soep							

welke extra frucht?

Figure 1 – An example of a dietary regime drafted by Alfred Vogel.

vrijdag 25.11.60

KLINIEK VOOR NATUURGENEESWIJZE „ROODE WALD"
NUNSPEET, TELEFOON K 3412-2281
ALLE CONSULTEN EN BEHANDELINGEN ALLEEN VOLGENS AFSPRAAK

12 uur

SLA:

GEKOOKTE GROENTE:

Aardappelpurée.

Hollandsesaus.

Groentegebak.

Yoghurt.

6 uur

havervlokkengebak
sinaasappel
soep.

andijvie
wortelen
rode kool
boerenkool.

biet.

s.v.p.:
geen boeken op leggen.

Figures 2 & 3 (opposite) – Examples of patients' daily diets at Rood Walde.

KLINIEK VOOR NATUURGENEESWIJZE „ROODE WALD"
NUNSPEET, TELEFOON K 3412-2281
ALLE CONSULTEN EN BEHANDELINGEN ALLEEN VOLGENS AFSPRAAK

maandag 5.12 '60

<u>12 uur</u>
Rauwe groenten:
Andijvie
Wortel
Rode kool
Koolraap
Boeren kool
gekookte groenten:
Bonen

Rijst
Kruidensaus
Groentegebak
Kwark
Tomatensap

<u>6 uur</u>
Fruitsla
Noten
Soep

religion or even husband or wife, but if you want people to change their diet, you have a tough job on your hands.'

When we worked together, he always took time to impress upon me the importance of the dietary aspect of any patient's treatment and stressed that this was the first thing that should be tackled. And I have found, like Alfred, that this is not always a popular approach. Over the years, I have received a lot of verbal criticism during my lectures when I have spoken on diet and dietary matters. I clearly remember one lecture, which was filled to capacity, where some men were standing at the back of the hall waiting for their wives. They started banging on the doors, shouting that I had to stop going on about my bl**** diets! I have often been subjected to people swearing and cursing at me when I try to convey to them the importance of the dietary aspect of daily living. This usually happens when I recommend that people give up something that they are particularly fond of.

Vogel was aware all those years ago about the detrimental effects that a bad diet could have on people's health but, once again, such valuable advice was not heeded. The result today is that levels of obesity in the Western world are at almost epidemic levels. Our children are getting fatter and fatter, as many of them are brought up on diets of convenience foods full of fat, sugar and additives. The level of allergies is increasing rapidly and the health problems caused by this situation are quite frightening.

Western governments are now making attempts to address the situation but it is like trying to shut the stable door after the horse has bolted. Here in the UK we are being bombarded with gimmicky programmes and books about diet, but people should be careful about the advice that they follow. Faddy diets should be avoided and instead people should find a sensible balanced eating regime, such as those recommended by Alfred Vogel throughout his long career to promote good health.

One condition for which diet is particularly important is multiple sclerosis and by considering two different methods of treatment for this disease, the benefits of using organic produce – another prescient recommendation by Alfred Vogel – also become apparent.

When I was an 18-year-old student in Holland, I worked as an assistant to a medical professor and one day I told him about a particular patient whose symptoms were puzzling me. After I had relayed the details of the case to the professor, he told me that he wanted to see this patient for himself. Although multiple sclerosis was practically unknown in Holland at that time – I had never before heard of the disease – following some diagnostic tests, he said, 'This is a typical MS case.' In those days, the only thing he could recommend to the patient was Dr Evers' diet. Dr Joseph Evers, a German physician, believed that many illnesses were due to artificial methods of producing and processing foods. He recommended that only unprocessed foods be consumed, such as raw root vegetables, wholewheat bread, cheese, raw milk, raw eggs, butter, honey and so on. Salt and sugar were banned, as well as leafy greens and certain vegetables such as rhubarb, asparagus and cauliflower. Vital to this diet was the daily consumption of germinated wheat.

When I later discussed the Evers diet with Alfred Vogel, he confirmed that he had noted some degree of success with patients who followed this approach, but as my career has progressed, this has proved a bit of a puzzle to me for reasons that I will now explain.

In the 1960s, I met a man called Professor Roger MacDougall, who had developed his own dietary methods of controlling the symptoms of multiple sclerosis. He had worked out his own regime after being told that he was suffering from the disease and that nothing could be done for him. The puzzle for me lay in the fact that the diets devised by the two men seemed to have fundamentally different principles. Roger MacDougall's findings were that gluten could cause inflammation on the myelin sheath – leading to problems with the conduction of nerve impulses – and should be avoided at all costs, while on the Evers diet, patients were advised to consume daily rations of wheatgerm – wheatgerm, of course, containing a fairly large amount of gluten. Both approaches were apparently successful to some degree in containing the disease and with examples like this, it is not surprising that people become confused when one person says they should eat this and another person says they should eat that.

When comparing the two diets, however, I found far greater success with putting patients on the gluten-free programme. And Alfred Vogel confirmed that in countries he had travelled to which had a very low rate of cases of multiple sclerosis, such as Japan and Iceland, the gluten intake was extremely low. But this still did not account for the fact that any success was noted amongst patients following the Evers diet and this is where the importance of organically grown produce becomes apparent.

I noticed that when MS patients ate normal bread grains purchased from supermarkets, their health deteriorated more rapidly. In contrast, the grains used by Evers in his diet were completely organic and freshly sprouted. Under examination, it becomes apparent that the gluten content is significantly lower in such organic grains than in the artificially boosted grains that we consume today, which have been subjected to artificial fertilisers, insecticides and pesticides. After testing both theories, I found that each achieved a measure of success, but I saw a quick deterioration from those consuming what I called 'artificial' grains.

This was also relevant when considering allergies (which can easily lead to multiple sclerosis). It was often observed when a patient had an allergy to wheat, it was usually because the wheat was not organic and that was where the problems lay.

Once again, Vogel had shown remarkable foresight with his views on natural organically grown foods. I remember about 20 years ago when he compared samples of food bought in a supermarket with produce from our organic nursery in Troon. He was greatly interested in the in-depth research that was being carried out at Auchincruive Agricultural College near Ayr and this inspired him to carry out his own investigations. When these tests were completed, it was remarkable to see how superior the organic foods were and how much richer they were in vitamins, minerals and trace elements than those from the supermarkets which were grown with the aid of fertilisers, insecticides and pesticides.

Vogel had strict control over his own gardens and it was not unusual for him to be heard shouting at his gardeners when they did not adhere to his totally organic processes. Anything with even a hint of a chemical smell was banned. It was fascinating to see the array of produce that Vogel grew in his own gardens – and also in ours when he came over to train our gardeners. He always seemed to be at his happiest when he was working outdoors.

Vogel was also ahead of his time in recognising that there might be a link between diet and behavioural patterns. This was an area that was also of great interest to me after I spent some time working in a psychiatric hospital while I was a student. After studying many of the patients, I was convinced that what they ate affected their behaviour. In particular, many of the patients reacted adversely to sugar and became hyperactive and disturbed after consuming any sugary food or drinks.

At the beginning of the 1980s, I was given a fascinating opportunity to conduct more research into this area when I undertook a study of criminals in British prisons. I wanted to ascertain whether violent behaviour could be traced back to poor eating habits. I was convinced that allergies to certain foods could trigger disturbed behaviour and was delighted when members of the prison officers' association were willing to let me conduct research inside their institutions. They were obviously hopeful that my research would help them find effective ways to maintain order. Vogel was most interested to hear of this work and I kept in close contact with him throughout this period.

My first study involved the inmates of a female prison. I asked these women to keep daily diaries of what they ate and I also asked them to keep a note of problems they experienced due to hormonal changes. It became apparent through these studies that some of the women were affected by the poor quality of the food they were eating. Their diet was high in animal protein and sugar, and the effect this had was to turn them into Jekyll and Hyde characters. Many of them had also eaten poorly before being sent to prison and in some cases their violent behaviour (some had assaulted or even murdered their partners) appeared to have been exacerbated by what they ate. After committing such crimes, many of the women were full of remorse, as they had acted completely outwith the bounds of their normal behaviour. It is my belief that it was their diet that caused them to lose control to the extent that they even attacked the people they loved the most.

Women are particularly vulnerable at certain points of their menstrual cycle and there are some well-publicised incidents of women becoming violent when suffering badly from pre-menstrual tension (PMT). Following a balanced diet is very important for sufferers of PMT, in order to avoid fluctuating blood sugar levels, for example.

In another institution, one of my subjects had committed a number of murders. After spending some time with him and learning about his dietary habits, I became convinced that his appalling diet had affected his mind so much that it had caused him to lose all control and exhibit extremely violent behaviour. In my opinion, his problems had started when, as a young boy, his mother would give him candy-coated chocolate drops or coloured sweets to keep him quiet when he had been naughty, not realising that this was only exacerbating the situation and making him even more hyperactive. By the time he had grown up, he had become totally addicted to chocolate and biscuits, and there were many things to which he had become allergic.

When I first met him, it was clear that he found it difficult to control his temper and he was also asthmatic. When I talked to Vogel about this man, he listed all the foods to which the subject could possibly be allergic and when I undertook tests, Vogel turned out to be absolutely correct. Before carrying out his last horrific murder, I learned that the man had drunk six cups of milky coffee (and he was allergic to milk), each cup had six spoonfuls of sugar, which made him extremely hyperactive, and although he did not normally drink alcohol, he had some strong drinks which had a high gluten content. He then ate half a loaf of bread (the tests also showing that he was very allergic to wheat). He then ate a lot of chocolate and became so high that he totally lost control.

I carried out similar tests on many criminals and, having built up a considerable body of evidence, I have repeatedly asked for more consideration to be given to dietary management in British prisons, and for prisoners to be taught what to eat and what to avoid. Not only would it be good for their general health but it would also certainly save the lives of many innocent victims. I have pleaded with many MPs at the House of Commons and with peers in the House of Lords for action to be taken on this matter but, on the whole, my words have fallen on deaf ears. Is it really so unreasonable for us to pay close attention to a good balanced diet when people's lives are at stake?

The first people on earth mainly ate fruit, vegetables and nuts, and, later on, added some goats' milk. This does not sound much but, nevertheless, one could do much with such a diet. Vogel was a pioneer in this area and even when staying at the best hotels, he would arrive with his packet of muesli under his arm and plenty of fruit or vegetables in his bag for his breakfast. During our many travels together, I often admired him as his case would be laden with his home-grown organic apples and pears, and while I often offered him a meal, he would usually prefer to eat his own produce.

He was never ashamed to make people aware of his strong beliefs, his healthy diet and his natural medicine. I had a lot of respect for him as he continued preaching to his audiences that if they did not pay careful attention to their diet, then their health would fail. Unfortunately, of course, even when you are speaking the truth it is sometimes difficult to get people to listen to you.

Chapter 6

The physician or therapist is like a mountain guide: he leads and shows the way, but he does not carry the patients – they have to make their way themselves.

Alfred Vogel

A tremendous crowd of people turned up for one of my lectures last year in Arbroath. The audience seemed engrossed as I talked about my chosen subject, 'How to be in tune with your body', and after they had all listened intently, there was a lengthy succession of questions. The final question, from a particularly astute gentleman in the audience, was, 'How would you deal with patients who were not willing to follow advice or could not see the point in their treatment, and how much effort would you put into guiding such patients?'

There is no easy answer to this question, although the situation that he described – in which patients ignore the advice given to them – is a familiar problem for all health practitioners. I found it was only possible to respond by giving various examples.

I told the gentleman that each practitioner, of course, has the same responsibility – to ensure that they give the best possible help and guidance to their patients. At times, however, it can be extremely difficult to get people to follow this advice, especially, for example, where dietary management is concerned. One often has to rely on one's power of persuasion and one thing that I really admired about Alfred Vogel was his ability to convince people to do the correct thing. When we talked to people, he would often say, 'It is not mathematics, it is common sense – start by looking at your lifestyle, then try to correct what is necessary.'

The man who had asked the question was, quite understandably, not satisfied with such a vague answer, so I then quoted the old adage that although you can lead a horse to water, you cannot make it drink. As Vogel said, and I quoted at the beginning of this chapter: 'as practitioners, we are like mountain guides – we can lead the way but we have no control over how people will react to the advice they are given; they have to make their own way themselves.' While it can be frustrating when people fail to follow the good advice that they have been given, this would not lead me to turn them away or to stop trying to help them.

Another problem encountered by practitioners arises when patients expect to see quick results. If this does not happen, and they have to wait a long time to see any improvement in their condition, they can often lose faith in their practitioner and lose the will to carry on with their treatment. When this happened with patients of Dr Vogel, he would acquaint them with the saying that an illness or disease usually comes to us on a horse but can leave us on a donkey – in other words, you need to have patience. When a patient has tolerated a longstanding illness for, say, more than a year, then it could possibly take a few years to be completely free of that particular complaint. As a practitioner, it is vital that you are able to convince your patient that you will be able to help them, as this is perhaps the only way you can persuade them to continue with treatment when they often feel like giving up.

I then illustrated this point with a story about one of the miracles that I have been fortunate enough to witness during my lifetime. This involved a female patient who had multiple sclerosis. As she was virtually unable to walk, she first arrived to see me in a wheelchair. I immediately gave her some acupuncture and recommended that she follow the gluten-free MacDougall diet. She returned to see me and, during her third appointment, as she was coming off the bench after the acupuncture, she told me she had a little more feeling in her legs and asked if she could try to stand. With my help, she was able to stand and, before leaving the clinic, she actually managed to take a few steps.

When she turned up for her next appointment, I saw her sitting in the waiting room and noticed that the wheelchair was missing. I asked my assistant to have a look to see if it was in the cloakroom but she returned saying it wasn't there. I then called out the name of the patient, Maureen, whereupon, remarkably, she stood up and walked with me to the treatment room. I asked her what had happened and she told me that she could not believe the sudden improvement after the many years she had spent practically unable to walk. Needless to say, her muscles had weakened during that time and, with multiple sclerosis, when the strength diminishes, it is most unlikely that it can be regained. When the myelin sheath is broken, it can rarely be healed, and what is dead is dead. But although this woman would never regain full power, she was able to walk again, even if it was with difficulty. Given the poor state she had been in when she first came to see me, this transformation in her condition was amazing.

I have been fortunate during my lifetime to have witnessed several successful cases of patients who have managed to control their disease through dietary management and this was clearly the case with my friend Maureen. She continued to do very well but then, without warning, she stopped coming to see me and I wondered if she was all right.

About three or four months later, she returned to the clinic, back in her wheelchair again. I asked her what had happened. She said she had tried to work it out for a long time. She told me she had been doing well until she paid a visit to her neurologist. He greatly discouraged her by saying the improvement she was experiencing would almost certainly only be temporary and all he could do for her was to arrange for a chair lift to be installed in her house. The following day, she was unable to walk.

Being quite religious, I told her some biblical stories about how Jesus had healed people, as I wanted to prove to her that the mind is stronger than the body and that the power of suggestion – either positive or negative – can be so strong that it would either work in her favour or it would be disastrous. She listened intently. The stories I told her were quite pertinent and she luckily understood the point I was trying to get across to her. I also recommended some additional soft-tissue manipulation. Thankfully, I managed to convince her to continue with the treatment and after a few weeks, she was able to walk again; a number of years later, she continues to do so.

Alfred Vogel had a special ability whereby he could motivate people to believe in themselves and to become aware of what they were capable of achieving to help themselves. I discovered this when my wife Joyce and I arrived in Teufen to study with him. I have already mentioned the rather cold reception we received when we disturbed him at his work but when we did eventually get to speak to Vogel, I found him inspirational. He made me believe in him, and in myself, and after that meeting I felt as though my whole life was undergoing a revolution. He was so convincing in his belief that one must be in tune with nature in order to be in tune with oneself.

When Professor Geers, a famous professor of geology, came over from Finland with a group of students, I went with his group into the Jura mountains to study with Vogel. It was an amazing trip during which I came to appreciate even more how closely Vogel lived to nature. He was able to identify all the species that we saw on our journey and describe the attributes of each plant and flower. He picked up plants with such tenderness, examining the way they were growing and explaining why the leaves grew from the stem. He was so knowledgeable about nature and this was also displayed in his research work, where he crossed different species of plants to achieve tremendous results. Not only was he in tune with himself but also with nature, and that special gift enabled him to produce the exact remedy he was aiming for. It was because he believed so passionately that he wanted to be like a mountain guide. He wanted to share his enthusiasm with others and point out all the beauties to be found in nature. He wanted to show people the way to make changes in their lives that would be of great benefit to their health.

In this he was similar to a Scotsman called Dugald Semple, who shared many of Vogel's philosophies. Semple was a loner who travelled from one place to another in his small horse-drawn caravan. He felt it was his responsibility to investigate the quality of the soil being used to grow plants and foods, and also to find out which chemicals were being used. He did so by working and digging in the fields around him. Like Alfred, he too had a message to preach and later on, when he had his own little property, he held lectures to try to encourage people to discover their inner strength and explained how this strength could be built upon. Although he was seen by many as being very eccentric, he did develop quite a following and he was very influential in the vegetarian movement in the UK.

Vogel also believed it was vital for people to find inner peace. When he held lectures, for example in London, he took advantage of every opportunity to tell listeners that they did not need to belong to a religious sect or a political party to find inner peace. It was something that everyone could discover within themselves and once they found it they could use this power to overcome many problems and obstacles.

During his lectures, Vogel tried to persuade people to live according to the laws of nature and he did the same with those people who came to visit him at his little clinic in Teufen. It was not an easy task to reach him on that mountain, far away from all the hustle and bustle. But life there was calmer and enabled him, as a guide, to show people how to find inner peace. It was then up to each individual whether they followed his advice or not. Throughout our work, Vogel and I continually emphasised to people the importance of following our advice carefully and persevering until their problems cleared up. Unfortunately, people can so easily lose faith and quickly be led astray.

As well as providing guidance for individual patients, Vogel tried to use his powers of persuasion to influence change on a much larger scale. As I have already mentioned, he was very concerned about the damage that Man was doing to the environment and he took every opportunity to highlight these problems to governmental bodies and international authorities.

He attended inter-governmental congresses on environmental matters and tried to impress upon the authorities the damage that was being done to nature and the problems that mankind was creating for the future. He asked people to take action and to do something about the situation. One particular congress sticks out in my mind, as Alfred made a notably impassioned plea. At this important meeting of the Swiss Association for the Protection of Nature in 1972, Alfred spoke so convincingly that he even succeeded in convincing one of the managing directors from the chemical corporation Ciba-Geigy that changes were needed to stop large conglomerates from harming the environment. His charisma really was remarkable.

At that same congress, another speaker highlighted an issue that was also of vital interest to Vogel. Professor Picard, the well-known French professor of chemistry, said that, on this beautiful earth that was entrusted to us, we have to do our best to safeguard all that is natural and warned that if we did not stop adding poisons to the foods we were consuming and adding rubbish to the soil to make produce grow bigger, then one day we would reap what we had sown.

This, of course, was a subject about which Vogel was passionate. He was terribly worried about the quality of food and constantly pointed out that while the artificially fertilised and treated produce on sale in supermarkets might be big and might look nice, it is of little benefit to people's health if it doesn't contain the correct vitamins, minerals and trace elements. Vogel worked tirelessly in his herbal gardens day and night to guarantee that high quality was reached and to give back to humanity what he felt he owed because of the life that he had been given. He was also conscious of his own mortality, wanting everything he learned to go on being of benefit to others, and he often said to me, 'One day I will not be here and it will then be up to you.' So, today, that responsibility lies on my shoulders as I carry on Vogel's hard work.

As part of trying to get the message across to the younger generation, I often invite them to accompany me when I confront governments or those people in charge to try and impress upon them the harm that is being done by the proliferation of all these chemicals in the food chain. As I said in a previous chapter, things have to be in balance. When a weighing machine is in balance, then its negative and positive are neutral. The same is the case with the cells in the body – but if we do things that adversely influence them, then those cells will become negative. We must therefore stop and think of the damage these harmful additives are causing. We are all born with cells of regeneration and degeneration but when the cells of degeneration (as in the case of cancer) rapidly take over from the regenerative cells, then problems arise. However, there is still a lot that one can do to regain that balance. The food we eat, the water we drink, the air we breathe: these are all important elements in helping to keep our cells in balance. As I have often pointed out, a cancer cell is an oxygen-poor cell, so it is therefore crucial that we strive for purer air and reduce the levels of air pollution.

As previously mentioned, Vogel also stressed the importance of adhering to a diet with a proper balance of carbohydrate and protein but he went further with his advice in this area. The optimum daily amount of protein is between 40 and 70 grams, and it is crucial that this is derived from the best source. It makes a vast difference whether we get our protein from a pig or a soya bean. The same goes for carbohydrates – if they are from the correct sources, then we will reap the benefit. Vogel tried to put this point across in many lectures and, as he was also concerned about the poor quality of bread being produced, he decided to make his own.

He was totally opposed to white sugar and used to warn about the harm that it would do to people's teeth. Vogel was always surprised to see that people from the West Indies had white, healthy teeth but although they had sugar in their diets, this was of the dark brown, unrefined variety. They extracted this fresh liquid, which they called 'pillo sillo' (this is how they pronounced it, I'm not sure how it would be spelled) from sugar cane. One problem today is the amount of hidden sugar in processed food and drinks. For example, a lot of sugar is added to processed fruit drinks, making them unhealthy. It is much more beneficial to drink freshly squeezed fruit juices.

Fruits are naturally sweet, so there is no need at all to add refined sugars to them. If we want to eat something sweet, then it should take the form of natural sugars from good-quality fruits, but at the end of the day, it is our choice whether we eat refined sugar or natural sweeteners, such as honey.

Even though Vogel gave this advice many years ago, and pointed out the problems that would arise if it was not followed, little notice has been taken and we are paying the price with health problems today.

I was very intrigued when Vogel once took me to a factory that produced a wonderful remedy called *Molkosan*, which is naturally fermented concentrated whey made from the residue of cheese-making. Not only is *Molkosan* a great antiseptic (which can be used in the treatment of such problems as verrucas and fungal infections) but it is also of tremendous help to diabetics in assisting with the production of additional natural insulin. It can also help weight loss, when taken together with kelp, as this helps to regulate the body's metabolism.

The process of making *Molkosan* is very complicated but it is one of the finest products prescribed by me on a daily basis. Once again, however, I cannot force my patients to follow my advice.

The problem with *Molkosan* is its slightly unpleasant taste. But people should be able to overcome this if they are aware of how beneficial it can be for their health. It makes a nutritious drink, and yet many people find it unpalatable. Each individual therefore needs to experiment to find a way of including it in their diet to suit their own individual taste. When combined with other ingredients, *Molkosan* makes a rich and delicious salad dressing, for example, or you could mix it with a combination of fruit to make up a morning drink.

I cannot believe how short-sighted some people can be. I decided to try and make this product in Holland to help overweight Dutch people, so I went to a factory with my bottle of *Molkosan*. I told the managing director that if he agreed to produce this on my behalf, then the number of people with weight problems in Holland would probably be reduced by about half. He smiled as he visualised the money already rolling in to his company and asked to try the product. As I handed him the bottle, I advised him not to taste it in its pure state but he proceeded to do just that. He was so put off by the taste that he refused to make it for me. So I went to another factory in an effort to find someone willing to produce this excellent remedy.

I eventually succeeded but when I see it on the shelves today and it is not sold as readily as it should be, I often think of the many people, like myself, who are obtaining great benefit from it. Being a diabetic, it has helped me to stabilise my condition without taking the medication that would otherwise have been necessary.

Molkosan is a wonderful remedy in the treatment of so many conditions and yet, if one does not search for the underlying cause of the problem, then one can never wholly treat it. Many times Vogel said, 'Pain is like an alarm bell. The body will tell us that something is not in order, but we then have to take a look at what is wrong. We cannot stop the clock or allow the problem to continue. We have to investigate matters and find the source of the problem.' Today, the big problem is that people are dosing themselves with drugs to treat the symptoms of their problem instead of getting to the root cause of what is wrong.

On one occasion when Vogel was visiting me in Scotland, he sat in on a consultation I was having with a local fishmonger. This man had been feeling very unwell for a while now and was experiencing difficulty with his breathing. He had been given various drugs by his own doctors but nothing had been effective and he was desperate for help. Although he didn't totally understand what the fishmonger was saying, Vogel turned to me and commented that the man had a lot of toxicity in his system and that he needed something to help him breathe, as he was gasping while sitting in the consultation room. Vogel suggested giving him four tablets of kelp a day and monitoring the situation. Sea kelp works like a sponge, by somehow helping to mop up the waste that is dumped in the sea, and kelp tablets help the body in the same way, mopping up some of the rubbish in our system and improving blood circulation, while the iodine it contains gives the endocrine glands a boost. It is also effective in controlling weight problems. We rarely see overweight fishermen, as even the smell of kelp will help keep their weight under control. I remember back in the 1970s, one morning while I was working at my clinic in Ayrshire, I received a phone call from a professor in Edinburgh, who invited me down to look at some sea kelp. It was fascinating, like a glowing mass.

The fishmonger followed our advice and whenever I met him after that, he always told me how grateful he was for the improvement in his condition. He said that he would never have believed that a simple kelp tablet was capable of giving him a new lease of life. The drugs he had been given by his doctor had been aimed at alleviating his obvious respiratory problems but they did not address the underlying problem of toxicity in his system.

As I have said, Vogel was very practical and learned a lot from the many people that he met. One day he took me out for a run in his big car. Like me, he was not a competent driver and the journey was quite stressful but, after some time, we eventually arrived at a farm where harvesting was taking place. Vogel knew this particular farmer and asked him to tell me what he did with the first cut of the harvest when it was brought in. The farmer told me that, first, he gathered together the tops of some of the oats and took them into the house, where some brandy or other alcohol was poured over them. The mixture was then stored in a cupboard and when his mother became a bit nervous or when his father was overworked, they would take a sip of this liquor. In homoeopathy, this remedy is called *Avena Sativa*, the Latin name for oats, and what a wonderful remedy it is, because the grains contain an ingredient called *avenine*, which is a marvellous tonic for the nerves. When discussing this remedy, I often think of my oldest patient who, at the incredible age of almost 108, has porridge every morning for breakfast. That is why she has such a wonderful nervous system – because she feeds her nerves with the oats in the porridge that she has made almost every morning during her remarkable life. Apart from those who are intolerant to oats, I would recommend porridge for breakfast to anyone. Unfortunately, however, it is not seen as being as tasty as the sugar-laden cereals that are regularly advertised on television, usually aimed at children.

Vogel also tried to spread his message through his lecture

tours or by taking part in radio and television programmes. When I joined him, I always admired the way he always seemed to have an answer ready for any of the questions that might be thrown at him. I particularly enjoyed it when he told the audience stories about the many discoveries he had made. On one occasion, he was asked a question about the importance of calcium. This was a subject which Vogel had studied very carefully and he told the story of his battle to obtain calcium in a form that the body would be able to assimilate. Calcium is one of the most important minerals in the human body. As most of us know, it is vital for our teeth and bones but less well known is the fact that it is important in helping our bodies to fight off infectious diseases. There had been various calcium preparations available for some time but none of these were particularly effective. Vogel had considered this problem over a number of years and he received inspiration from a well-known chemist that he met in Davos in Switzerland. This man had experience in producing calcium milk but was searching for a better way to deliver the benefits of calcium to the human body. He was utterly convinced that this would be possible and his conviction inspired Vogel to continue with his research. He looked to his beloved plants for the answer and finally succeeded in his quest. Today, in my own country of Holland, *Urticalcin*, which was the successful formulation, is one of the most frequently prescribed calcium remedies.

One of the plants that was most helpful in this preparation was the stinging nettle. Vogel knew what a wonderful plant the nettle, *Urtica*, was for a range of ailments, including anaemia, rickets and respiratory diseases, but one day he realised that

that if he mixed *Urtica* with calcium, then it would enter the bloodstream more quickly. What an excellent remedy he had produced and what a friend I have had in this preparation over the years in my practice.

With his incredible knowledge, Vogel wanted to impress on me that, as a practitioner, we have a duty to help people in more ways than one – not only by what we prescribe but also by leading and showing people the way through sharing our life experiences. The responsibility then passes to the patients to do as much as they can to help themselves with the advice we impart to them.Whenever he had a problem with his feet due to travelling or from standing too long, he would walk barefoot in the meadows. The healing properties of the earth always helped him, and he was never embarrassed to be seen doing seemingly unorthodox things, as he loved being outside with nature.

I remember one day when he asked us to do some translations for him after returning from having spent a few days in the Engadine. He had slept in the mountains overnight because he could not find anywhere suitable to stay. He did not believe in staying in upper-class hotels, as he was a man of simplicity. He would prefer to sleep outside in nature than somewhere that possibly wasn't clean and tidy or was too expensive. He also disliked staying anywhere with concrete or artificial flooring, as he said that they 'block the assimilation of cosmic energy'. He claimed that a cat or a dog will seldom lie on a concrete floor, even if covered by a blanket for them to lie on, and pointed to the example of his big black Newfoundland dogs. He told me that they would not go into the laboratory to sleep at night but were much happier to lie outside, even in the

91

snow, or on natural stone floors. They never lay on concrete floors, as they intuitively knew it was not good for them.

He never pampered himself with life's luxuries and, like myself, loved simplicity. That was one of the reasons I was so much in tune with him and that we worked so well together, as we were both on the same wavelength.

Vogel was ahead of his time in so many ways and he tried through various methods to spread his ideas to as many people as possible. But he was also aware that you cannot force other people to adopt your ideas or follow your example. Sadly, as life today grows ever busier and more stressful, people have less time to listen to what their bodies are telling them and look for solutions in nature as Vogel advised.

Chapter 7

My home is our planet.

Alfred Vogel

One of the many things I miss about Alfred Vogel now that he is no longer with us is his stories. He had so many anecdotes about the memorable events he experienced during his lifetime and his experiences during his extensive trips all over the world. I paid particular attention to those from the 1950s before we met. Later on, I was often lucky enough to accompany him on his travels and it was always a most enlightening experience.

As Vogel was continually on the lookout to discover more natural and traditional remedies, this tireless traveller journeyed throughout the world to further his knowledge of the age-old healing methods used by the indigenous people he met. He was always eager to visit museums and study people's lifestyles in an attempt to establish a link as to why in certain countries some diseases were virtually unheard of, while in others they were rampant.

He put a tremendous amount of energy into his travels and always liked to talk about his adventures at sea when he went to countries like North America in the days before air travel was widely available. He enjoyed experiencing the different climates and studying the soil of each country. I remember after I had been on a trip to South Dakota, I mentioned to him the volcanic soil that I had noticed. I knew that Alfred had travelled to that area previously and he told me that when he smelled the earth there, he realised that this wilderness had existed long before people started to discover it.

It was in the 1950s when he was visiting a remote part of South Dakota that he met a Sioux medicine man called Black Elk. This man introduced Vogel to the wonders of nature in that area of the world and Vogel was fascinated to discover how long the trees that he could see had been growing there. Most importantly, Black Elk also introduced Alfred to the power of *Echinacea purpurea*, which was a plant well loved by the Native Americans. They had a mutual respect for nature and forged a friendship which Black Elk sealed by gifting a handful of *Echinacea* seeds to Vogel. Vogel took these back to his herb garden in Switzerland and nurtured them. Then he studied them carefully and, as we have already heard, *Echinaforce* became one of his most successful remedies.

He would talk to the old medicine men of the tribes about their traditional methods of treating human suffering, the secrets of which had been handed down from father to son. He considered the Navajo Indians to be a very healthy group of people and believed that this was due to their use of herbs. They had a clear philosophy and maintained the traditional forms of medicine that had been handed down through the generations. He was interested to learn what foods these people ate and discovered that their diet was almost totally vegetarian; he also learned how they baked their bread and tried to establish what their average age was as a way of gauging how healthy they were.

Sadly, over the past few decades the lifestyle of these people has changed dramatically due to the encroachment of the modern world and its effects on their diet and the amount of physical activity that they undertake. In 1997, the US *Journal of Nutrition* published data from the Navajo Health and Nutrition Survey study which showed that 22.9 per cent of Navajo adults age 20 and older had diabetes. Fourteen per cent had a history of diabetes and another 7 per cent were found to have undiagnosed diabetes during the survey.

I remember, during lectures, that Alfred referred to a meeting he had had with an old Sioux Indian who was 118 years old, and how four generations of his family lived together in one small hut. With sadness, he would tell the story of how the white people sent the Sioux Indians into the wilderness where they were forced to work like slaves.

He also learned a lot from the Papagos Indians when he visited Arizona and was amazed at the fantastic array of herbs that they grew and the way they made use of these herbs to eradicate insects. He commented that the Papagos were attractive people who had a very healthy lifestyle.

During the years 1950 to 1952, he lived for a short time in Pipeline Avenue in Pomona, California, where he learned a great deal about acupuncture, reflexology and other methods of treatment. While there, he became friendly with the well-known actress Gloria Swanson, who wrote a number of articles about his book *The Nature Doctor*, which was first published in 1952, remarking that every household in the United States should have a copy of it.

He also lectured at several colleges in the area on chiropractic, osteopathy and naturopathy but, after a while, felt he wanted to travel further. So, next he headed to Iowa.

When he arrived there, he saw enormous towers of corn being doused with petrol and set alight. When he asked the farmers why this was happening and why they did not seem to be concerned that their crops were being wantonly destroyed, they told him that they were being given large subsidies by the government as they were, in fact, growing too much corn. Vogel was appalled by this. He thought it was an absolute disgrace for perfectly good food to be destroyed in this way when there was so much hunger in the world. He was so annoyed that he wrote to Congress and the Senate and managed to make some headway with them, the burning being stopped at that time. He was always very friendly and open and had a positive outlook. Even during his darkest experiences, he kept a clear vision and even when confronted with problems such as a sandstorm in Nevada he was never discouraged from travelling.

I always had the feeling that he had a great love for Mexico, as he spoke warmly of the wonderful time he had spent there. When talking about the native people, he would say, 'As long as you remain friendly, they will be open and tell you what you want to know.' His passage through the country was not always easy, though, as people could be very suspicious of strangers. In the village of Lagos de Moreno, for example, he encountered problems with the head of the village, who thought he was a

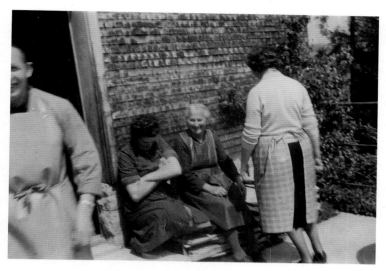

At Teufen in the early days.

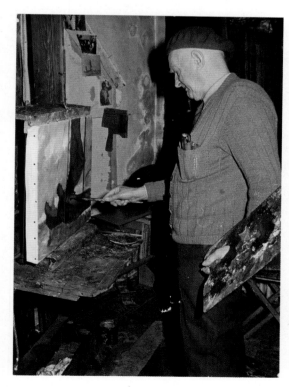

My great friend Joss Lussenburg, who greatly enjoyed his discussions with Alfred Vogel.

Bioforce going upwards.
The company was
founded by Alfred
Vogel in 1963 and
continues to thrive
today.

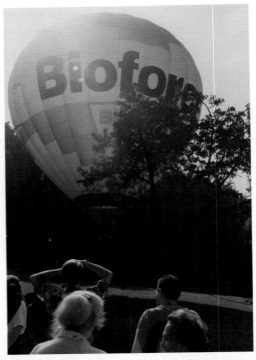

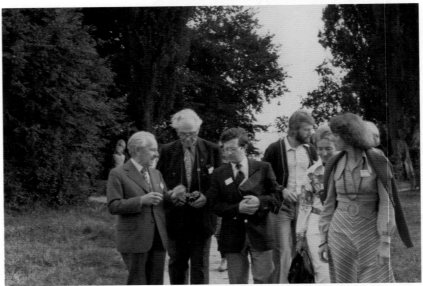

With Professor Geers, the tallest man in the Swiss Alps.

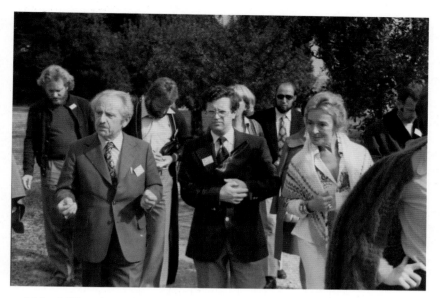

Alfred Vogel explaining the use of herbs in the Swiss Alps in the 1970s.

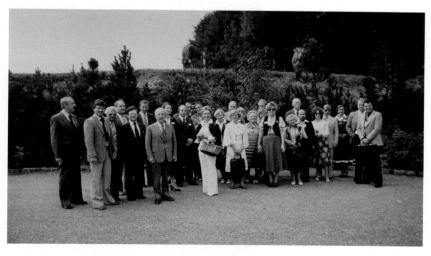

Alfred and his co-workers in the 1970s.

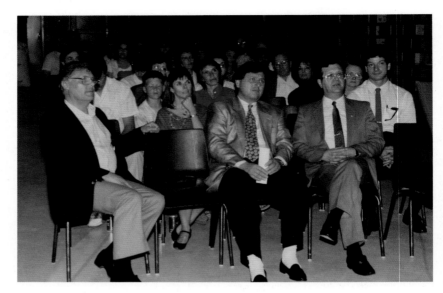

Mr Geiger, Claus Smidt and myself
listening to Alfred Vogel in Canada.

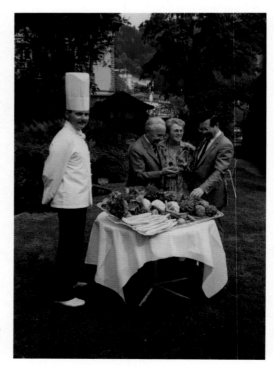

Alfred and me looking
at some healthy foods.

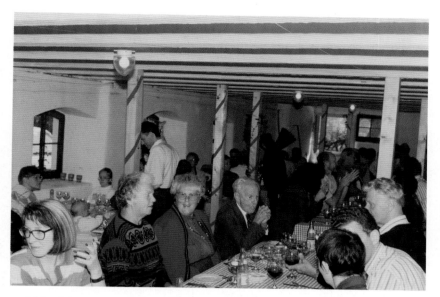

Alfred having a healthy dinner with his second wife, Denise, and his daughter, Ruth.

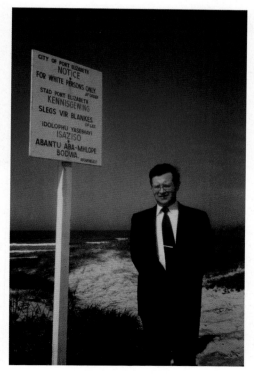

I travelled all over the world with Alfred Vogel and I was shocked by the evidence of apartheid in South Africa in the 1980s.

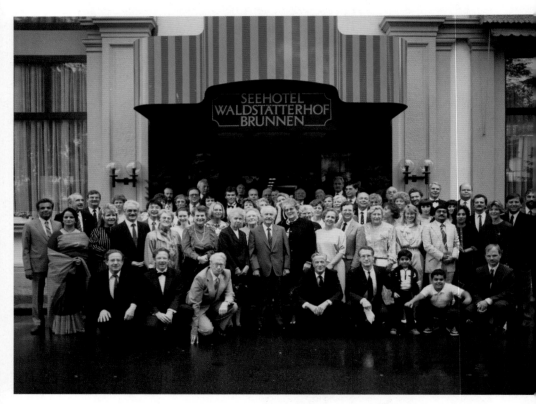

Alfred with some of his co-workers in 1985.

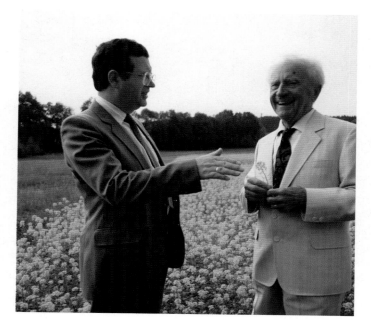

We both agreed how important it was to maintain
a positive attitude and a good sense of humour.

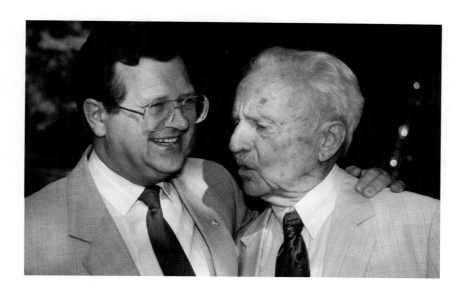

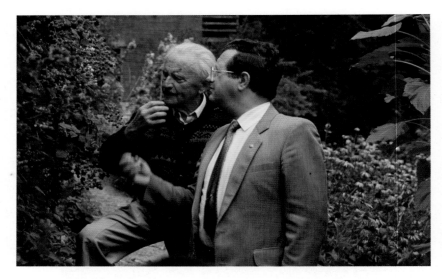

Alfred and me examining some *Cratageus* berries.

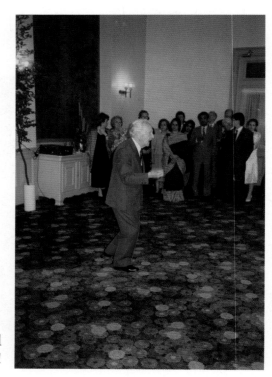

Alfred in his 90s – still
very active!

spy and wanted to imprison him. Alfred's wife, Sophie, and his daughter, Ruth, became so distressed that they clung to Alfred and pleaded with this leader to let him go. All three then started to sing some old Swiss songs as a way to try to show these people that they were not a threat. Luckily, as Vogel could speak Spanish, he was eventually able to convince them that he was a Swiss naturopath, not an international spy, and they let him go.

Another memorable experience Alfred had in Mexico was his visit to the gardens of Xochimilco, where he walked around the herbal gardens and inspected the beauty that nature had to offer. When he showed me some photographs he had taken, I could see what a wonderful place it was. In Mexico City, he realised again there was a lot to learn from people in different countries as he studied their metabolic therapy method of treating cancer.

During some lectures, Alfred would talk about Guatemala and I can remember him advising people that if they wanted to eat honey, then they should choose Guatemalan. According to him it was the purest available, as it was free of insecticides and pesticides. The Guatemalan people, especially those from the Ministry of Agriculture (MAGA) were very friendly, and in the east of the country, he spent some time with a Swiss family, which he thoroughly enjoyed. In 1976, Vogel was very upset to hear of the horrendous earthquake that had devastated Guatemala but he was relieved when he received news that his Swiss friends had not been badly affected.

After Guatemala, he then travelled through Colombia and Ecuador, where he carried out a lot of good work, and when he arrived in Peru, he was so impressed by the country that in 1958 he bought a farm where he proceeded to grow potatoes, bananas, cherries, papayas, etc. He sold these to the local people at the markets and he used the herbs that he grew to produce his remedies. Not only did he toil barefoot in these fields himself when he was able to visit the farm but the local Peruvians also helped him tremendously. In turn, he helped them with his research and application of *Tormentil Complex* to help with common bowel problems that the people were suffering from. He also used *Molkosan* to help combat the effects of poor hygiene.

He travelled extensively throughout Peru during his visits there, making the most wonderful videos and taking spectacular photographs. He thought it was such a beautiful country and loved to go down river on expeditions. One story which I will always remember was about an Indian tribe who had built their huts out of tree trunks. He tried to converse with them as best he could as they sat around a small fire. He learned how they would pound the poisonous barbasco root and, when this substance was put into the river, the fish would come to the top, gasping for air, thus enabling the fishermen to easily scoop them up. They would then cook the fish, often in the liquid from palm trees and citrus fruits. It was quite amazing how tasty they were and how, in this remote part of Peru, people were very healthy.

One thing he never discovered was how the Indians of South America prepare curare. They used to coat the tips of their arrows with this substance and, using their bows, would fire them at their enemy or prey. Curare produces paralysis in muscles. In fatal doses, death is caused by respiratory paralysis.

Although Alfred managed to get a small jar of it, he never actually found out what exactly it was made from.

He had some near escapes during his travels and I remember the story he told about one plane journey through the mountains in Peru when they suddenly flew into a dense blanket of cloud. The pilot of the very small 16-seater plane was forced to skilfully guide the plane above the clouds but at this altitude the oxygen levels in the tiny craft were greatly reduced. Although the passengers were sick and felt miserable when they eventually landed in Cusco, there was also great relief that they had managed to land safely. Luckily, Alfred had some *Crataegus*, *Echinaforce* and *Ginseng* with him and managed to help the passengers by administering these remedies. He always took *Echinaforce* with him wherever he went and, if he came across any problems, he would use it to help the local people, especially with any skin or bowel problems.

From Cusco he travelled to Machu Picchu, which is a remote settlement perched high in the Andes mountains on a steep-sided ridge. He was amazed by the remains of the ancient Incan civilisation that had been discovered there at the start of the twentieth century and felt that it was a very spiritual place.

He learned so much from the people and the plants in South America, and it was with tears in his eyes that Alfred told me that he had been compelled to sell his farm in Peru after the government legislated that outsiders were only permitted to own 15 acres of ground.

When he travelled to Africa, he wanted to find out what illnesses were prevalent on that continent and also about how the diet, which he believed to be high in protein, affected people's health. He did a lot of research there into problems affecting people's kidneys, lungs and bowels, and also into infectious diseases.

I remember how enthusiastic he was when he returned home in 1973 with some *Harpagophytum* (*Devil's Claw*), which he had discovered on meeting the Ovambo tribe in the wilderness in Namibia. I have often written about how these people used *Devil's Claw* as we would use potatoes and Vogel personally witnessed the tremendous benefits to those people who used this plant daily. They obtained all the natural mineral salts they needed from this source and even although they lived in conditions similar to a sauna, they still had no kidney problems or rheumatism. Vogel brought this plant back to Europe, where it has been used to treat, among other things, fevers, skin lesions, gout, rheumatoid arthritis and conditions affecting the gall bladder, pancreas, stomach and kidneys. When in South Africa, he held a lot of lectures on the healing properties of herbs and plants. He was very interested in the Dutch and Germans who had settled in that country.

In addition to the aforementioned countries, he also travelled to Israel, Jordan, Lebanon, Syria and Iraq several times, and he accumulated a lot of facts about the people living there and their history. He talked to the Muslims about their beliefs and, while travelling in the mountains, he learned a lot about people's attitudes, their clothing and their lifestyle. He was interested to find that as there were no refrigerators, the people in these areas used olive oil extensively as a preservative for their foodstuffs.

I was fascinated when he told me about the mountain he

climbed, Mount Nebo in Jordan, where Moses died. It is my opinion that Moses must have been the greatest leader ever to have lived because, for a period of 40 years, he led the Israelites through the wilderness so that they could enter the Promised Land. Alfred had visited the place where Moses ended his tremendous journey and I was eager to hear all the details of this trip.

In Lebanon, Vogel was particularly keen to see the Cedar trees there that were over a thousand years old. He was surprised to see how healthy the Druze people were, particularly their strong teeth. He was fascinated to witness how these people lived and was excited by the culture of the Middle East.

He also travelled extensively through India, Indonesia, China, Taiwan, Thailand, Korea, Japan and the tropics. He witnessed many problems in the tropics, which prompted him to write his invaluable book on tropical diseases, which, as I mentioned earlier, is now an invaluable addition to my own library. He also visited institutes of tropical diseases to share his knowledge on the different methods that people could use to treat these conditions and to stress the importance of good hygiene.

In Thailand, he was very interested in the rice-growing process, and always believed that brown rice from Thailand is the finest and most beneficial for one's health. He took careful note of the diets of people in the various countries that he visited, notably of the bread and cereals that they ate, and many of these products are luckily now available throughout Europe. Once again, he stressed the importance of achieving balance and pointed to nature for an example. In Thailand, he witnessed how one animal will kill another to keep nature in balance, as exemplified by the many snakes he witnessed killing the rats and mice that were destroying the rice fields.

In Korea, he was particularly interested in the ginseng found there. The Koreans use not only the root of the ginseng but part of the plant itself in order to maintain a strong nervous system. This is the perfect illustration of Alfred's belief that it is sometimes necessary to utilise the whole plant to obtain the optimum benefit.

During Alfred's lectures in countries such as Holland, Germany, Switzerland and also America, his listeners were always captivated by the stories of his exotic travels. I remember one time when we were in the United States when he talked about his magazine, *Gesundheits Nachrichten*, which continues to be published today and to which I have contributed a lot of articles. On this occasion he spoke about one of his own articles, in which he wrote about Ceylon (now Sri Lanka), where he came across many people with elephantiasis, a grotesque hardening and thickening of the skin which was particularly prevalent in people who lived around Mount Lavinia. Elephantiasis occurs when the sufferer has become host to parasitic filarial worms that lodge themselves in the lymphatic system. Female worms release millions of microfilariae (immature worms) that circulate in the blood and the disease is transmitted by mosquitoes. At one point during their trip, his daughter started to present signs of this condition and it was amazing to see how *Echinaforce* helped her overcome it. As a result, he recommended it to the local people and whenever he travelled to Sri Lanka, he often made use of that particular remedy. During his many travels, he often came across dangerous situations and diseases, so Vogel always went prepared!

During his lectures, he repeatedly spoke about the

importance of life and when he spoke about the suffering that he had witnessed or the way that Man was destroying nature, he would often have tears in his eyes. For example, he always became upset when he thought of the tragic events that took place in Hiroshima and Nagasaki, and how, as a result, people there are still dying of cancer and leukaemia.

Alfred often said that being interested in what is happening around the world keeps you young. I try to follow his example and I shall always treasure the things he taught me following each excursion. Alfred thoroughly enjoyed his travels and this is why he so often said, 'My home is our planet.'

In his book *The Nature Doctor*, Vogel relates a lot more about his travels, but the ones I have mentioned here are those that are special to me. It is with the greatest joy that I think of the journeys we made together, mostly in Europe, and what we learned from the beneficial remedies that we came across, many of which I have written about in this book. It is wonderful to think that this small man shared his great knowledge so as to help alleviate human suffering. From the days of his youth, through his many travels, his one aim in life was always to help people. He managed to do this not just through his clinics, but also through his magazines and then the huge factories that eventually followed to produce the remedies that he devised.

Chapter 8

Each plant is complete in itself; it proceeds from a formula based on intelligence, forethought and wise planning. The precious value of the individual plant is jeopardised if its delicately balanced structure is torn apart. Every substance contained in a plant has purpose and significance. They complement each other and act as a whole.

Alfred Vogel

On my last visit to Holland, I was taken to see some *Echinacea* plants that were growing on what was once the floor of the sea. The Dutch have made a great achievement by reclaiming land from the sea and in doing so have made available some of the most fertile soil in Holland.

The fields that I was looking at belonged to our company Biohorma, which Vogel and I established in 1972. This is the Dutch arm of the parent firm Bioforce, which is based in Roggwil, Switzerland. Bioforce was established in 1963 to enable the manufacture of Vogel's remedies on a larger scale.

The majority of plants used to produce Bioharma products are grown on site, allowing us to maintain complete control over the cultivation of the plants – from planting to harvesting – and ensure that Vogel's principles are still applied today. As the company was continually expanding, it became necessary to reclaim land and these areas proved to be particularly suitable for the cultivation of herbs.

As I stood in the middle of that field of *Echinacea* plants, my mind wandered back many years to the day when we opened the first clinic for natural treatments in Holland, and to the many obstacles we faced in importing the remedies that we prescribed. The bookkeeper came to me one day and said, 'Jan, we cannot expand any further. Importing goods from Switzerland has become so costly that the products are too expensive to sell.' Taxes were rising and transportation costs were escalating to such a level that we had to consider alternatives. We managed to persuade Dr Vogel that my wife, Joyce, and I should go to Switzerland to become skilled in the processes involved in making the remedies and, thereafter, return to Holland and put our newfound knowledge to good use by making the same products there. I have already given a brief account of that period in my life in the first part of my autobiography, but I would like to expand on this a bit further now.

When we arrived in Switzerland in 1961, we received a great deal of support from Dr Reinmalt and the then general manager, Mr Metler. Those two gentlemen possessed the same dedication and precision as Vogel himself but my greatest admiration was reserved for Alfred, whose knowledge in this

field was second to none. I was amazed at how intelligently he
had concocted those medicines. He had recorded all the

Blasenschwäche	Blasentropfen
	Urticalcin
	Cina D 6
	Wallwurztinktur innerlich &
	   äusserlich
	Sitzbäder in Absud von
	   Spitzwegerichtee

Blattern, spitze	Echinaforce Lachesis D 12 Viola tric. D 1 Molkosan zum Betupfen Urticalcin-Pulver z. Bestäuben Johannisöl z. Betupfen

Bleikoliken: Bleivergiftung
 bei Buchdruckern
	Opium D 3) über
	Natrium sulf. D 3 - D 6) längere
	        ) Zeit ein-
	         nehmen

Blinddarm-Reizung	Lehmwickel event. Johannisöl trinken

Blutarmut (Anaemie)	Alfavena
	Urticalcin
	Galeopsis
	event. Chelicynara
	  Ferrum phos. D 3
	  Arnica D 3
	bei grosser Schwäche: Avena sativa
	      Arsenum alb.
	         D 4
	Darm reinigen
	viel grüne Salate, Brennesselsaft,
	sehr viel Spinat, Gemüsesäfte,
	      Rüeblisaft,
	in Rotwein eingeweichte dunkle,
	gedörrte Birnen
	hin und wieder ein rohes Ei in
	Traubensaft verschlagen,
	rohe Randen, Randensaft
	Alpenkräutermalz

Figure 4 – Recommendations from Alfred Vogel
for the treatment of various diseases.

formulae in a large ledger, which he kept with him at all times, and I have illustrated here an example of one such creation.

The combinations that he blended, added to the detailed advice he provided to treat each illness, were remarkable and of great benefit to so many people. He always ensured that he obtained the total picture of a patient's medical history and lifestyle before starting to combine remedies to suit their individual needs.

During our lessons, we learned how important it was, when we were making the tinctures, that everything was correct, right down to the smallest detail. The Swiss were meticulous and everything had been taken into account in each stage of the production process. Close attention was paid while growing the herbs, after which the factory workers macerated them with the greatest care through the final processes until the remedies were produced. I always felt proud when the Americans said they considered these remedies to be the Rolls Royce of herbal medicines. Many have tried and failed to reproduce them. Vogel's techniques were in tune with the natural products he was working with and that is what he tried to pass on to me. The following information from Bioforce UK explains a little bit more about the processes involved:

Holistic Standardisation is the process by which we ensure that every batch of Bioforce herbs is as potent and effective as it should be. We look at every ingredient within the plant and test each batch of herbs to confirm that the full spectrum of ingredients is present to the necessary level. This process differs from Chemical Standardisation, whereby one component of the plant is selected as being responsible for the action of the plant, and only the levels of that one component are measured. Bioforce believes that every element within a plant contributes to its overall effect and should be present in a tincture in the amounts found in the original herb.

We worked extremely hard during our visit to Switzerland and were fortunate to receive a lot of cooperation from the staff. We also went into the mountains with Vogel to widen our knowledge of the plants and herbs.

When we returned to Holland, we were able to start manufacturing some of the plant-based products, although, initially, only on a small scale. We realised that we were taking a big step but, as someone said to us, 'You need to start somewhere and people who have the courage to start will reap the rewards once the process becomes established.' Thankfully, after we entered into a legal agreement with Vogel for the recipes in his ledger, we had all the formulae we needed to get this new venture off the ground.

As the business expanded, we moved to Elburg. Under the management of Mr Bolle senior, things ran more smoothly and, together with my previous colleague, Mr Arie Drenth, we were able to open a manufacturing plant. Today, that has grown into Biohorma as we know it.

As my mind returned to the field of *Echinacea* plants, and I looked at those vast buildings and fertile fields, I was filled with pride at developing this important business. It was not without hard work, though. There were many times when. things were extremely difficult and everything seemed to be

BETERSCHAP

AMERIKA	AUSTRALIË	BELGIË	NEDERLAND	DUITSLAND	CANADA	ZWITSERLAND
565-35th Avenue	29 Ghelnsford Ave	25 Rue Henri de Saegher	BIOHORMA	Vogel & Weber	1188 Berristreet	Bioforce
San Francisco-Cal. USA	Epping NSW	Bruxelles 8	NUNSPEET	München	Montreal-St. N.	Teufen AR

Hulp uit Zwitserland

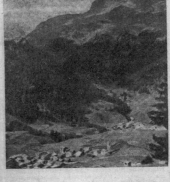

Loop niet door met uw klachten

Dank zij de medische vooruitgang in de laatste jaren is het sterftecijfer van tuberculose, kinderverlamming en verdere infectieziekten sterk gedaald. Wat een steeds groter aantal artsen nu grote zorg baart, is het ontstellend hoge cijfer chronische patiënten, dat ondanks hun harde werken niet daalt, maar integendeel nog dagelijks toeneemt.

Natuurlijke hulpbronnen

Astma, reuma, bloedsomloop- en spijsverteringsstoornissen zijn maar enkele van de vele plagen. De pijnen en directe ziekteverschijnselen kunnen wel bestreden worden, maar het ziektebeeld zelf blijft praktisch onveranderd. Met een gevoel van wanhoop vragen vele patiënten zich af of er niet méér gedaan kan worden om te helpen.
Natuurlijk kan er meer gedaan worden!
Kruiden hebben al van onheuglijke tijden af genezing gebracht. Oude kultuurvolken kenden aan kruidendranken, die bereid waren door kundige handen, hoge waarde toe.

Verbluffende resultaten

Zij die reeds lang geplaagd worden door een aandoening, kunnen blij zijn dat er nieuwe mogelijkheden voor hen zijn. Laboratorium Biohorma te Nunspeet importeert namelijk de Zwitserse kruidentinkturen van ▓ A. Vogel. Deze geneesmiddelen hebben internationale bekendheid gekregen, mede door de vaak verbluffende resultaten. Alleen al in Duitsland zijn er honderden artsen die ze geregeld voorschrijven. In de korte tijd dat deze geneesmiddelen in Nederland en België verkrijgbaar zijn, hebben zowel artsen als patiënten ze leren waarderen.

Waardevolle adviezen

Vele ziekten vinden vaak hun oorzaak in kleine voedings- en levensfouten. Iedereen die een kuur van Dr. A. Vogels geneesmiddelen bestelt, ontvangt daarom in een begeleidende brief uitgebreide medische adviezen. Deze zijn geput uit de grote ervaring die ▓ A. Vogel en buitenlandse artsen hebben opgedaan. Eenvoudige waterbehandelingen, het al of niet eten van bepaalde voedingsmiddelen, enz., ondersteunen de goede werking der kuur. Vanzelfsprekend zal een en ander geschieden in overleg met de huisarts.
Dit zal nu werkelijk een hulp zijn voor mensen die misschien al lang de hoop op beterschap hebben verloren.

Hoe groene planten u kunnen helpen

De Zwitserse natuurarts Dr. Alfred Vogel, één der grote kruidenkenners van onze tijd, is van mening, dat men niet ongestraft chemische geneesmiddelen in het lichaam kan brengen. „Het lichaam is geen chemische fabriek", zegt Dr. Vogel in zijn door duizenden gelezen blad „Gezondheidspost". De enige juiste manier om een ziek organisme te helpen is een beroep te doen op de natuurlijke hulpbronnen die in duizenden kruiden verborgen zijn.
Wanneer men, zoals meestal de gewoonte is, kruiden na het oogsten droogt en in pakhuizen opslaat, gaat er veel van de natuurlijke geneeskracht verloren. ▓ Alfred Vogel laat de in het wild verzamelde kruiden direkt koud uitpersen en het genezende groene sap wordt dan één van de kruidentinkturen. Dit koude bewerkingsproces is mede oorzaak van de hoge geneeskracht van deze kruidengeneesmiddelen. Door oplettend en nauwgezet te werk te gaan, kunnen alle natuurlijke hulpbronnen voor de patiënt behouden blijven.

Zwitserland, vindplaats van waardevolle kruiden

Geneeskrachtige kruiden worden hier verzameld op een hoogte van 1600 - 2500 meter. Ze groeien weelderig op de vaak steile berghellingen. Zwitserse kruiden bevatten méér geneeskracht, omdat ze profiteren van de natuurlijke bodem en intensere zonnestraling. Ervaren verzamelaars zoeken de plantjes in de tijd, dat ze net volgroeid zijn.

Kruiden brengen genezende werking

Figure 5 – The front page of the first edition of *Beterschap* (Health News).

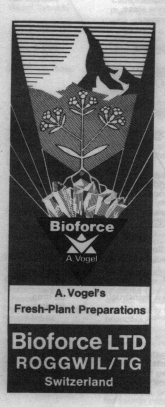

Remedies from nature

Wandering in sumertime through the Bernese Highland, along the foot of the Matterhorn, or in the many side-valleys of the Engadin, yes, even upon the heights of the limy Jura we come upon a colourful flora of various herbs, many of which are well-known, proven medicinal herbs.

But not only in our country, in far off continents as well, in the highlands of the Andes of South America, in the tropical jungle of East Asia there plants are growing the curative effects of which are useful to mankind.

Since antiquity, the herb-medicines derived from them belong to our faithful helpers.

A. Vogel, the well-known Specialist for Phyto- and Nutritiontherapies, brings into full view to you some of his proven herbal remedies which – wherever possible – are prepared from fresh plants. The preparation is carried out in the new, up-to-date factory of the BIOFORCE LTD., in Roggwil TG. Your special shop where you will receive this prospectus will be pleased to let you have further information. Allow Vogel's fresh-plant preparations to become your helping friends. By these quite a number of health troubles can be removed.

In case of need we are recommending you the following products which have been well proved for many years.

Bioforce
A. Vogel

A. Vogel's Fresh-Plant Preparations

Bioforce LTD
ROGGWIL/TG
Switzerland

BIOFORCE

Figure 6 – This was one of the first brochures that we produced.

against us. Favourable publicity from magazines such as *Beterschap* and leaflets such as 'Remedies from Nature' (of which I have illustrated the first pages) brought our work to people's attention and, from then on, our business expanded greatly and is still going strong today.

The *Echinacea* plants at which I was staring with such pride, were, of course, descendants – if that is the right word – from those seeds given to Vogel by Black Elk all those years ago in South Dakota. The Prairies of America are a long way from the foothills of the Swiss Alps, but it was in those Alps that Alfred Vogel tended Black Elk's seeds in the wholesome soil and healthy fresh air at his Teufen clinic. Those seeds, so carefully husbanded all those decades ago, provided the foundation for the now glorious fields of those wonderful purple-headed stems which grace the Bioforce fields in Switzerland and Holland. Each is still carefully sown and gently harvested as Vogel always wanted.

When I looked at those *Echinacea* fields on reclaimed soil in Holland, that story – along with many others spanning the long number of years I shared with Vogel – came to my mind. If he ever discovered a plant of which he had limited knowledge, then he would think about its possible characteristics and signature before extensively researching it. As his work continued, so the pharmacy of natural herbal medicines in that little place of Teufen flourished.

Vogel had initially found it difficult to acquire arable land of the highest quality in Switzerland so I was delighted when in 1963, full of pride, he told me of some ground he had found that was of exactly the standard he was looking for. He felt it was like a gift from heaven, as it was well known that the likelihood of acquiring land in that area of Switzerland was remote.

The memory is so clear in my mind when I think back to that special day when he took me to see the wonderful new place in Roggwil where, in perfect peace and tranquillity, the medicinal herbs continue to be cultivated today according to Alfred Vogel's principles. As he stood there, he asked, 'Did you ever imagine that things would have expanded to this extent?' and he told me about the negotiations he had had to go through to acquire the land and continue with his quest to help his fellow human beings. You could see how humble he was about how he had managed to get everything to come together. His great desire was to offer people more help in their fight against illness and disease and to repair what Man had destroyed so easily.

When Vogel started his work he was fortunate to be able to have a lot of freedom in the remedies that he prescribed. Nowadays, our work is restricted by red tape and there is a proliferation of legislation outlining what practitioners are and are not allowed to do. People in authority have withdrawn some of the most valuable remedies from the market, which were more beneficial than many of the prescribed drugs with proven side effects. Sadly, their interference has not been in the best interest or well-being of the public but geared more towards increasing the profits of the giant drug companies. In contrast, Alfred Vogel was an individual who always put his patients' welfare first.

It is a great worry to me that, in today's society, the world is heading in the direction whereby people care more about money and materialistic possessions than for their fellow human beings. My grandmother was a wise old lady. At the age of 98, as she lay on her deathbed, she took hold of my hand and that of my cousin, who was a matron in a hospital, and said, 'You have both been called to help people. The biggest enemy you will face in the world will be the selfish attitudes of people who become lovers of themselves.' Vogel disliked such people. His compassionate heart always went out to those in need.

When he visited us in Scotland to offer advice on running our clinic, I often wondered if any of the patients realised what a brilliant man was in their midst. I remember one occasion when I was attending to a patient who was in a lot of pain Vogel took off his jacket and started to work on this man using an old German practice called *Baunscheidt*. This is a very rigorous treatment and involves puncturing the skin with needles and then pouring oil over the area, which becomes very red and inflamed. It was invented by a German mechanic in the nineteenth century as a counter-irritation measure and it seemed very effective in relieving this patient's discomfort. Vogel told me of the people he had treated using such old, established methods in instances when patients had difficulty walking or were completely immobile. In cases where people had become totally lame and modern medicines did not offer any answers, he would turn to those old methods. He sometimes achieved the most amazing results by using the seemingly bizarre technique of rubbing bulls' testicles into the spine!

During one of his visits, when we held a lecture in Ayr, he selected a few people in the audience who were really ill and tried to offer them some guidance. He had that intuitive gift of being able to sense those who were unwell and to be able to talk to them with compassion. He focused on one particular lady, who was almost crippled with rheumatoid arthritis, and said to me, 'You have to treat this patient. You have the same gift as I have, and that is the gift of intuition. You will know how to treat her.' I went on to take care of that lady for quite a number of years, during which time she improved greatly. She said to me, 'Wasn't it a blessing that I was at that meeting and that Alfred Vogel picked me out and brought me to you, so that I now no longer need my wheelchair but can walk.' Instances like those make my work worthwhile and make me more eager than ever to continue.

I can recall one consultation I had with a 12-year-old girl while Vogel was visiting. He listened carefully to our consultation and I noticed he had tears in his eyes as he sat in the corner. Alfred realised that, as she had a very aggressive form of cancer, there was very little hope for this girl and her young life would soon come to an end. With deep compassion, he spoke to her and her parents and offered some advice to make things easier for them all. He shook his head when they left and said to me, 'It would be wonderful to think that one day illness and untimely deaths will be a thing of the past.' I have always admired the loving attitude of that great man who worked diligently, harnessing the forces of nature, to help his fellow human beings and, indeed, together we worked hard to ease people's burdens. Until the day he died, he was completely true to these principles.

Today, Vogel's philosophies have come much more to the fore, with many of his ideas being replicated and a lot of his views being repeated. His favourite remedies are still sold worldwide and I am sure that he would have been proud to see the 'A. Vogel' name on them today – not only those that he worked on totally by himself but also the ones that we worked on together.

Seeds from cultures. This guarantees us the greatest possible genetic uniformity.

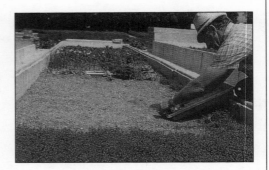

Cultures are planted according to biological principles. The use of chemicals is replaced by the expensive use of manpower: weeding, composting and manual harvesting.

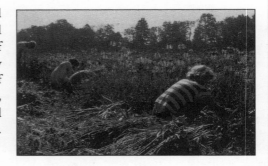

From planting through to the finished product, constant checks and laboratory analyses help to ensure the quality of our products.

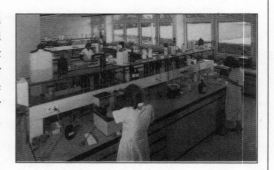

Figure 7 – The process of making Echinecea.

Chapter 9

In all your striving, let love be your guide for it is
the greatest power in the universe.

Alfred Vogel

Quite a number of years ago I accompanied Vogel to New
York, where he addressed an audience in a large packed hall.
He spoke on a variety of subjects and ended the evening on a
very unusual note by quoting the words above.

He told his listeners that we were living in a world that had
become so selfish we had no consideration for the welfare of
our fellow human beings. To emphasise this point, he
mentioned the biblical story of Cain and Abel. When Cain
murdered his brother Abel and God called him to order, Cain
asked, 'Am I my brother's keeper?' It is that spirit that Vogel
warned us to beware of in the modern world, and it is certainly
one that is unacceptable to those who believe in God. In every
walk of life, God demonstrates his greatest love. When we look
at the universe and all that He has created, we come to realise

that love is the greatest power and will be the strongest force in achieving peace.

That lecture was actually held not far from the site of the appalling disaster of 11 September that took place many years later in 2001. When I heard of that horrific tragedy, I thought back to the words spoken by Vogel that evening. I realised that people had learnt nothing from the story of the beginning of creation, or the devastating events of two world wars that destroyed the lives of millions of innocent people. It is regrettable that we have not learnt that lesson to love each other and to realise that we *are* each other's keepers. A conscious effort must be made to help each other in this troubled world of which we are all a part.

I remember when I travelled by train with him and his wife, Denise, from Newcastle to Glasgow during one of their visits to the UK. As he looked at the sheep peacefully grazing on the mountains during our journey, he started to tell me about the benefits of sheep eating certain herbs that were freely growing there. He then repeated one of his favourite sayings, 'In nature, everything is in balance.' He looked sad, however, as if thinking about what human intervention was doing to upset that balance.

During that journey, I told him a little about the history of Hadrian's Wall and how the Roman soldiers had built it to protect the northern boundary of the Roman Empire from hostile tribes that then inhabited Scotland. It is astonishing that sections of that wall are still visible and accessible today, which is a testament to the builders' skills. As a good road system made it easier for the emperors to control their empire by being able to send messages and orders more quickly, the roads had to be well constructed and straight. Excellent examples of these straight Roman roads can still be seen in the Newcastle area today.

Vogel agreed what a mighty empire it had been in its day. He then asked me, 'Do you know what caused the fall of that mighty Roman empire?'

I replied, 'Yes, I do know. They lost their empire as a result of immorality.' He informed me that, many times during his lifetime, he had seen how important and famous people had lost the battle with immorality. It is important that we keep our lives on a straight path. As he was a man to whom 'yes' meant 'yes' and 'no' meant 'no', he was as straight as the Roman road to Newcastle.

We discussed the importance of keeping order in life and about the tremendous hatred and jealousy that taints the modern world. He acquainted me with the story of an Indian prince who marvelled at one of his fellow believers – a poor man who, in spite of his poverty, rejoiced in the prince's wealth and his graceful wife. When the puzzled prince questioned him, the poor man happily explained, 'Why should I not rejoice in beauty, especially if it does not occasion me any worry or responsibility? You have the burden of overseeing all your wealth and of providing for all your wife's needs, while I, on the other hand, can rejoice in just looking at your treasures without any worry.' In *The Nature Doctor*, Vogel said, 'Those who can enjoy the good fortune of others without feeling envious have passed their first big test which will ensure them happiness and peace throughout their lives.'

Vogel always looked at the positive side of things and remained optimistic even in the face of some very negative situations, such as when he had been deceived or people had taken him for granted. Many people in life tried to imitate him. Many tried to copy some of his wonderful recipes and his philosophies, and even went so far as stealing some of his possessions. He never complained much about it, though, and on the contrary, would remark, 'As long as it benefits other people.'

Vogel and I concurred that sharing is one of the most rewarding things in life. As with Vogel, I have often come across dishonest people and have had things cunningly taken from me but I really believe that those people who steal will never prosper. Being honest in life will not only benefit oneself but others as well. You reap what you sow in life and that is possibly the only justice there is.

He devoted a great deal of time to each individual who was in need of help. I remember a lecture he held in Zwolle, a city close to where I was born in Holland. A small man who came to chat to Vogel after the talk was so influenced by what Vogel had said that he sat down and cried. He told Vogel that his life had amounted to nothing and he explained that he could never be forgiven for the many sinful things he had done. As so often happens in such instances, his great sense of guilt had affected his physical, mental and emotional health. The things that we do wrong in life, or the dark secrets that we keep, all have a detrimental effect on our well-being. Guilt, jealousy, hatred and selfishness are some of the negative emotions that can gnaw away at our normal healthy existence.

Vogel spent a lot of time counselling this man and explained that forgiveness is unending. He said it could be compared to the sea, which was so vast that his sins, in comparison, would be forgotten about. He tried to lift the man's spirits by offering him advice and explained what an enormous help *St John's Wort* (*Hypericum perforatum*) could be to him. In addition, he prescribed some *Avena sativa* to calm his nerves. He suggested that he should ask for forgiveness and repent, and then start his life anew. The man replied that his life was so dark that he could not see any glimmer of hope but Vogel reminded him that behind every dark cloud there is sunshine. He directed him to put the past out of his mind, to look forward, be positive, to get his health back on track and then start over again.

It is an awful situation to be in when you cannot see the light at the end of the tunnel. Thankfully, however, it sometimes only takes a small event in life to lift one up and turn things around, so that we have the strength to carry on and start a new life. That man looked much happier as he said goodbye to us and I realised that I had learnt yet another lesson from my old friend, this time in how to offer guidance to people who feel they have come to the end of the road – it was another example of how Vogel tried to be his brother's keeper.

I shall always remember when I said goodbye to Alfred Vogel for the last time in this life. I spent a wonderful day with him in his home in Switzerland. Even although I could see that the end of his life was approaching, I was astonished at how sharp his mind was. We reminisced about some of our experiences, the different countries we had visited, the advances in what we refer to as 'complementary medicine', the changes that he had witnessed during his lifetime in people's lifestyles and society in general.

We were able to look back on many important achievements

They are carrying on his work

Alfred Vogel's "ambassadors" throughout the world

Nowhere else in the world have the thoughts and philosophy of Alfred Vogel fallen on such fertile ground as in the Netherlands. "The Nature Doctor" alone will soon have reached a circulation of one million copies, thus becoming one of the most widely read Dutch books of all. Alfred Vogel's ambassadors are particularly active here, with specialist courses, a visitors' centre and the

"Alfred Vogel Prize", awarded every five years for scientific contributions in the service of natural medicine. The ideas of Alfred Vogel are also being propagated in many other countries by delighted patients who pass on their positive experiences to others, as well as by doctors, heads of clinics and research workers.

"Alfred Vogel's contribution to our understanding of medicinal plants and their effects has been outstanding", explained Dr M. O. Bruker, the internationally renowned doctor and head of a respected clinic for holistic medicine in Lahnstein, Germany. Recently, at the final session of a conference of the Society of Medical Advisers Dr Bruker introduced Dr Alfred Vogel to the delegates in the following way: "He has always argued passionately for a reawakening of an awareness of the forces that lie within nature. In long, steady work with his patients, the readers of his journals and books and the audience at his lectures he has defended the use of medicinal plants and argued for a return to a simple lifestyle close to nature. Today, he is in a position to note with satisfaction that he is no longer a lone voice in the wilderness."

Dr Bruker, who has been a supporter of Alfred Vogel's for decades, is known to the public for his many scientific publications in which he has demonstrated, above all, the links between the "diseases of civilisation" and a diet and lifestyle that has become unnatural. Nowadays, among doctors, the significance of Dr Bruker's knowledge and experience for the future development of medicine

is being recognized more and more.

The message of the advantages of a lifestyle and of a medical treatment in harmony with nature is also making itself felt in teaching and research. In Germany there are already some chairs of natural medicine at universities. In Switzerland the necessary political moves have been taken in Bern and Zürich, and similar efforts are afoot in other countries. Dr

Silvio Jenny, long-serving head of the Bircher-Benner clinic in Zürich, commissioner for the professorial chair in Natural Medicine in Zürich and President of the Swiss Society of Practical Medicine said at a recent conference, in the presence of Alfred Vogel, that it was time to undertake "a further step towards the integration of plant medicine in modern medicine." Phytotherapy, as it was represented by Alfred Vogel, had limits set

by nature. Within these limits, however, there was still an extremely extensive area for research and discovery. Because of this, felt Dr Jenny, the discipline of phytotherapy had to reclaim its rightful place in the medical system.

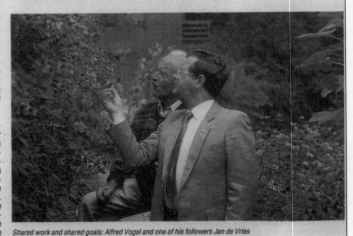

Shared work and shared goals: Alfred Vogel and one of his followers Jan de Vries

Figure 8 – Vogel's work attracted worldwide interest.

that we had made and I told him that I had recently seen a patient whom I had previously discussed with him. This girl had been suffering from cancer and had been told by conventional doctors that nothing more could be done for her, but I was delighted to report that, thanks to the advice he had given, she was now very happy and healthy.

This patient also represented another great achievement – as the wonderful methods he had researched and developed had now gained the respect of many orthodox practitioners. I don't think I ever witnessed a prouder moment in Vogel's life than when I handed him a letter written by an eminent consultant from one of London's foremost hospitals, who asked, 'What did you do to make this girl better? You have certainly accomplished something that we could not do.'

Science is a wonderful thing. We cannot survive without knowledge but, in so many situations, common sense is also necessary. This girl was probably examined scientifically from every angle and, yet, the scientists and conventional doctors had forgotten that she was just like any other human being – a part of nature. If she was ill, it was because there was an imbalance in her body. So, where did the imbalance lie when I first saw this girl? After delving into her medical history, I was able to piece together where the problems lay. Love and compassion were required to understand where she had been so misunderstood. First of all, her physical, mental and emotional bodies had to be put back into balance. We prescribed different remedies, examined her diet and also offered her counselling – and these sensible treatments made it possible for this girl to regain her health.

Even when we faced a barrage of criticism and

misunderstanding of our work, I always said to Vogel that we owed it to mankind to carry on. It can be very difficult to continue to strive to do one's best for others in the face of hostility and contempt but it is always worth it in the end. If we possess love and compassion, and if we tackle life's problems with some common sense, then hopefully we will be rewarded by success, as was certainly the case with our work with this girl.

Vogel was very happy that day as I left and, knowing that it would be the last time I saw him on this earth, I was comforted by the fact that he knew in his heart that he had done his best. The love and compassion that he had demonstrated to his fellow human beings during a lifetime of hard work and dedication had definitely paid off.

Chapter 10

There is nothing common about common sense.
Jan de Vries

One day when I was in Dublin, my eyes were drawn towards some bookmarks that were on sale in a bookshop. Imprinted on them was the above inscription, followed by my name. I never knew that these bookmarks were in circulation, although I regularly use that expression in my lectures. My parents taught me this lesson while I was growing up and I have applied it many times in life. Common sense is vital, especially in the approach to good health or in looking for answers to life's uncertainties.

I recall one particularly difficult, tiresome day when Vogel and I had had to face a barrage of unforeseen problems. It was not until we were leaving work and Vogel said to me, 'I really don't feel like doing this lecture tonight,' that I realised how much the day had drained his energies. That was very uncharacteristic of Vogel, because he never allowed anything to beat him. Even in his advancing years, he was always eager to tackle a problem head on. Looking at me, he then continued, 'I think you should take the lecture tonight.' This rather surprised me and I replied that it would not be the proper thing to do, as the hundreds of listeners who would be attending the lecture that night were going there to listen to *him* – not me.

I decided to try and lift his mood by telling him an amusing story about Albert Einstein. On his final lecture tour, Einstein apparently told his chauffeur that he did not want to do a particular lecture, just as Vogel had revealed to me that evening. His chauffeur, who had a white moustache and bore a close resemblance to the famous physicist, said, 'I shall do it, Professor. I have listened to your lectures so many times that I know them off by heart.' Amazingly, Einstein agreed to this unusual arrangement.

The lecture in question was being held at the Institute of Science in New York. Einstein decided to sit inconspicuously behind a pillar at the back of the hall to listen to his chauffeur. The chauffeur actually delivered the lecture very well, until it came to the moment where the audience could ask questions. As students like to grill guest speakers, a very difficult question was put to him. The chauffeur looked at the undergraduate and ingeniously replied, 'You must be a fool. Even my chauffeur who sits at the back of this audience could answer that question.'

Well, there was great hilarity in the car as I told Vogel that story and it appeared to cheer him up a great deal. I said to him, 'We may both be small but I don't have a moustache, and even although we do look like each other in many ways, I would definitely not be able to fool the audience into thinking I was you!'

When we arrived at the lecture hall, I asked Vogel if he was feeling a bit better. Although he said he was, he added that, because he was tired, he was going to deviate from the usual routine of his lectures. As it transpired, the lecture that followed that evening was the best he had ever given, although he never repeated it.

He started by telling his audience that, although he was there that evening to speak to them, he wanted to spend the time with them answering their questions. I actually wrote all those questions down and happened to come across them while I was writing this book. What amazed me about his answers was that a lot of them were basic common sense. I would now like to share some of them with you.

One of the first questions was, 'How long do you need to take the remedies for?' Vogel replied by wisely stating that, ideally, the body should be able to look after itself and should be allowed to repair itself. It is only when some extra help is needed that medicines should be used. Remedies for acute problems such as colds and flu should only be taken for a limited period – to give the body a boost. People who have a low immune system can benefit greatly from taking such remedies as *Echinacea* and *Urticalcin* to help increase their protection against ailments. But these remedies should also only be taken for a short time, then stopped for a spell before restarting if it is felt that a further boost is needed. With conditions like multiple sclerosis and rheumatoid arthritis, the remedies would probably have to be taken continually, though, of course, each case would have to be looked at individually.

As I have said, common sense is required. Women who are experiencing physical symptoms associated with the menopause, for example, can gain welcome relief by taking *Salvia* and then discontinue it once their symptoms have either subsided or disappeared completely. In the case of fungal infections, however, it can often take a long time before they are brought under control and it is sometimes necessary to keep taking particular treatments for a prolonged period. In these instances, Vogel stressed how important it is for people to be patient and to believe in the remedies they have been prescribed. He repeated one of his favourite phrases about illness coming to us on a horse and leaving on a donkey, and stressed that patients should consult their practitioners rather than stopping a remedy when *they* feel they should.

I came across such an instance not so long ago with a patient who had been consulting me about her rheumatoid arthritis. She was actually progressing well and, because of her improvement, she wanted to stop taking the remedies I had been prescribing. I asked her if she had any financial concerns that would prevent her from continuing the treatment, to which she replied, 'No, but I want to stop.' I advised her to keep taking them for a little longer, because her condition would most probably improve even further. However, she did not heed my advice and, when I met her three months later, she was almost crippled and begged me to take her back as a patient. All those months previously, I had advised her to keep taking the remedies as I wanted her to be well again, but she failed to use her common sense and pay attention to my advice.

Another question that was quite interesting was, 'Is it safe for pregnant women to take these remedies?' Vogel said something that I always emphasise to pregnant women, 'Please be very cautious when pregnant, as you should not take anything unless you absolutely need it. Talk to your doctor, practitioner or midwife and make sure that you read any labels thoroughly.' If there is any risk at all, then the labels usually warn against taking a particular remedy during pregnancy, but it is crucial that women pay extra attention in such instances.

During that lecture, a small, crippled lady stood up and asked a question relating to rheumatism and arthritis. Without delay, he asked her if she was anaemic, but she did not know. Unlike me, Vogel had never studied Chinese facial diagnosis and I could see that her facial expressions definitely revealed the outward signs. When she came to speak to us at the end of the lecture, I gently pulled her bottom eyelid down and said to Vogel, 'Here is the evidence of a tired, listless, anaemic person. We need to help her as much as possible.' We did so by giving her vitamins, minerals and homoeopathic remedies.

Then another man stood up to ask a question about his health and I smiled to myself as, straight away, Vogel asked him if he owned a castle. He looked rather puzzled and replied that he did not. 'Well,' said Vogel, 'the "walls" around your eyes show that you must live in a castle. The very first thing we need to do is to break down those black walls under your eyes. It is possible that your kidneys need some attention.' The man asked Vogel if he had second sight, to which Vogel responded in the negative. He then asked if there was anything that could be done so that his kidneys could perform their job more efficiently. Vogel started by enquiring if he was fond of salt – to which he replied that he loved salt and that the salt cellar was never far away from him. The first bit of advice Vogel gave him was therefore to reduce his salt intake. He then recommended that he drank plenty of water – not sparkling mineral water, but good clear water – and, with the addition of some *Solidago Complex* and *Golden Grass Tea*, the 'walls' around his castle would soon disappear.

A lot of questions were asked that particular evening on the issue of dietary management. As I've already made clear, Vogel was a true campaigner for a healthy, balanced diet and he was a wonderful advertisement for the benefits of such a regime. At the age of 92, he bought himself a new pair of skis so that he could glide more quickly over the Swiss mountains – at the time he told me that vegetables and fruits (especially salads) were his favourite foods and he believed that if he didn't eat those things, he would not be able to participate in his favourite sport.

A lot of people asked what his main recommendation would be for a healthy diet and I was happy with the response he gave. He said he believed in an individual diet for each individual person. That is something I have always advocated. His main suggestions were to eliminate as many additives, E-numbers and artificial colourings as possible from the diet; to eat a lot of wholegrain products, rice and fresh fruit and vegetables; and to be sparing in the consumption of animal protein – soya, as an alternative, would be preferable. Care must also be taken with the three 'Ss' – salt, sugar and saturated fats. These fats should be eliminated from the diet and replaced with cold-pressed fats, such as olive oil, safflower oil and sunflower oil.

It is essential that greater emphasis be placed on increasing the consumption of alkaline foods and limiting the intake of acid-forming foods – this became evident when I was approached by the Dutch Health Service to carry out double-blind trials on patients suffering from arthritis and rheumatoid arthritis, in order to prove the efficacy of integrating alternative and orthodox medicine. These trials were also monitored by one of the universities in Holland and, at the beginning, I felt that the rheumatologist who headed the orthodox side of the research was negatively disposed towards complementary medicine. He often asked me bluntly why I was hassling patients to adhere to the diet I was giving them. But, once again, I was applying common sense in recommending a diet that would lower the acidity in their bodies and I was able to prove the benefits of my recommendations when the results of most urine samples from these patients illustrated complete over-acidity in their bodies. When this acidity was eliminated from their systems, the participating patients from my section were given a lot of relief from their pain.

Gout, for instance, results from an overabundance of uric acid in the body. Eventually this uric acid crystallises and settles in the joints, resulting in swelling, inflammation and unbearable pain. A diet that is more alkaline than acid can only improve the situation. Other conditions, such as arthritis, rheumatism, eczema, psoriasis and duodenal and peptic ulcers also develop from an overly acidic diet, so it is an important issue to address. In the trials, it was demonstrated that the patients who followed my dietary regime had more long-term success in treating their conditions than the patients treated by orthodox means who were given strong drugs. Although the conventional approach did work quickly to alleviate the symptoms of pain and inflammation, it did not address the root of the problem and so these patients remained crippled. It is therefore a matter of common sense to follow the correct diet in order to achieve long-term relief.

The foodstuffs that lead to the creation of acid in the body include meat (especially anything from the pig), cheese, citrus fruits, coffee, tea, alcohol and nicotine, whereas vegetables, fruits and even potatoes are more alkaline-based. Another benefit of cutting out acidic foods can be to lower one's cholesterol level – so it is certainly worth trying out these new eating habits.

Another question asked that evening was, 'Can eating a lot of raw food cause stomach problems?' Common sense again prevailed as Vogel explained that not only do raw foods (such as salads, vegetables and fruits) contain the most vitamins, minerals and trace elements but they are also rich in enzymes which aid absorption by the digestive system. Of course, however, if one suddenly starts to eat a large amount of raw food when the body is not used to it, this might cause a stomach upset. It is only sensible when a decision has been made to change one's diet, to do so gradually in order to allow time for the stomach to adapt.

Other tips that Vogel gave were to eat slowly and chew your food thoroughly before swallowing. Whenever you experience acid reflux or problems with indigestion, make a conscious effort to chew your food extra thoroughly, so that the saliva (which is your best aid in the digestion of foods) can mix with it, thereby assisting the process.

It was also stressed, in response to a few questions, how

imperative it is to ensure that recurring problems are investigated, and never to be concerned about going repeatedly to your doctor if you are at all anxious. As Vogel said, 'Your doctor should be your best friend, as he has a responsibility for your well-being.'

Chapter 11

Questions lead to wisdom.
                                        Jan de Vries

As I mentioned in the previous chapter, a lively discussion unfolded during an evening lecture when Alfred Vogel answered a series of some interesting and unusual questions that were put to him by an attentive audience. Although I had listened to him countless times and, in my 40-plus books, have written extensively about the many ailments that afflict people, because that particular evening was so memorable, I felt it would be a good idea to highlight some more of the issues discussed, as those queries are similar to the ones on people's minds every day. As I have often said, questions lead to wisdom.

One question came from an elderly lady who stood up and said that every single night, after just a few hours' rest, she would waken up and could not get back to sleep. Consequently, when it came time for her to rise in the morning, she was so sleepy and tired that she felt unable to cope with the day's events. Her doctor had prescribed sleeping tablets but she commented that these made her feel like a zombie.

Vogel replied that there were many reasons why people might have difficulty in getting to sleep or experience irregular sleeping patterns. He said that if people waken up at roughly the same time each night, then this may be as a result of tension, worries, drinking caffeine-laden beverages (such as coffee or cola drinks), sleeping during the day, lying on an uncomfortable mattress or eating a meal too late at night. He even commented that watching an exciting television programme just before going to bed could stimulate the mind and keep people awake. His advice was to try not to have a nap in the afternoon, to go for a walk in the evening and definitely not to drink alcohol, tea, hot chocolate or coffee at night, although a cup of bamboo coffee would be an acceptable substitute. Drinking this half an hour before retiring, with a spoonful of honey added to it and 25 drops of *Valerian Hops* can often rectify sleeping difficulties.

On the same theme, another lady stood up and asked how she could wean herself off sleeping tablets. She explained that she had been prescribed them for years and when she tried to come off them, she had difficulty sleeping and experienced other symptoms such as palpitations and heavy perspiration. Vogel informed her that, although sleeping tablets might have a calming effect, as they are basically tranquillisers, they contain ingredients that influence the central nervous system, which has a knock-on effect on other parts of the body. To take a drug like this can give rise to many problems. It can especially affect the endocrine glands and sometimes the lymph glands, where waste material can lodge. He urged her not to stop taking this medication suddenly but to gradually reduce the dosage. In the meantime, to help alleviate any withdrawal symptoms, she could take some natural alternatives. He also suggested that she either went for a walk or perhaps a cycle ride in the evening; or, if she had a dog, she should take it for a walk before going to bed.

Looking rather embarrassed, the woman then told Vogel that she had an irrational fear of going out of doors and asked if there was anything he could recommend that would help her to overcome this phobia. Vogel advised her to take the remedy *Avena sativa*, which has a restorative action on the nervous system, and not to give in to the fear but instead strive to overcome it. He recommended that she went out with a friend who could offer her support and, each day, to go a little further away from her home. He tried to offer reassurance by saying that the feelings of panic she experienced would gradually lessen until they no longer troubled her. He also suggested that she took some herbal remedies, such as *Ginsavena*, which is of great help in such circumstances.

The manager of a large company asked the next question. He had tried to get extra sleep but found it impossible unless he smoked several cigarettes before going to bed. He continued by saying that, although he had tried to stop, he was unable to sleep without them. Vogel informed him that, in dealing with any addiction, it takes approximately three weeks for the palate to become accustomed to the elimination of the addictive substance. He stressed to this man that if he could abstain from smoking for that three-week period, then he would most probably be over the worst of any withdrawal symptoms. He acknowledged that the first few weeks would be difficult but if he also examined his diet to ensure that he ate healthily, this would make things a bit easier for him. He was aware that a great deal of effort would be needed but said that the end result would make it worthwhile. He recommended he take five drops of a homoeopathic remedy called *Tabaccum* twice daily, and boost his diet by eating foods rich in calcium, magnesium and sodium. It was a pity that, at that particular time, I did not have the necessary knowledge of acupuncture, because I have helped many people to quit smoking using this therapy. This has been confirmed by the many testimonials I have received from people telling me how their health and lives in general have been greatly enhanced since they stopped. There is so much pollution in the air caused by smokers; I always tell them they were not brought into this world with a chimney on their head!

Another excellent question put to Dr Vogel was, 'Is it a responsible act to carry out self-doctoring?' When I look in shop windows or browse in shops, I feel that there is a remedy for everything and, as a lot are available without prescription, one can often treat oneself. I liked Vogel's answer because he said that there is no need for anyone to go to a doctor with everyday ailments such as nasal catarrh or a cough. As simple problems like this have been alleviated with remedies at home for a great number of years, then this is perfectly safe. However, it is always advisable to consult your own doctor when problems do not clear up, or if they recur. He said that one has to be cautious when self-doctoring by not taking over-the-counter medications for too long a period and to seek your doctor's advice if symptoms persist.. He also gave some examples of when medical attention should be sought immediately, such as for continuous coughing, coughing up blood, an ulcer that does not heal, difficulties in swallowing, a lump in any part of the body, blood loss, change in stools or pain when going to the toilet, difficulty in emptying the bladder and a whole host of other symptoms.

During this part of the discussion, someone asked why homoeopathic doctors and naturopaths are so against antibiotics. It is accepted that antibiotics are necessary in some situations and, as Vogel admitted, some antibiotics can be a real salvation. But one should not take them like sweets, as has been the case for many years in the Western world. The problem that arises through the overuse of antibiotics is that the bacteria they have been developed to combat become resistant and the drugs are therefore no longer effective. We are seeing the frightening results of this situation today with the spread of superbugs such as MRSA. It is also common for antibiotics to disturb the bowel flora, as they kill the good bacteria that aid digestion as well as the bad bacteria causing the infection. If an infection does appear, then you must consult your own doctor. The benefit of taking a natural antibiotic, like *Echinaforce*, is that the white blood cells increase but it does not attack the good bacteria in the bowel. If it has been necessary to take antibiotics it is advisable to take *Milk Thistle Complex* or *Acidophilus*, as these will help the bowel to recover. The questioner seemed quite satisfied with Alfred Vogel's response to his enquiry.

Another lady, in her 80s, said she had taken antibiotics for a considerable period of time and was now left with a tremendous noise in her ears. She wondered whether this could have been caused by their long-term use. Vogel said that there are four major causes of tinnitus – an ear infection, fungus, a vertebrae problem or congestion – and great care has to be taken to avoid this condition leading to deafness. If one also suffers from attacks of dizziness and severe nausea, then Ménière's disease may be the diagnosis. One can do a lot in such circumstances with the use of acupuncture and also by taking the excellent remedy *Ginkgo biloba*, which stimulates the circulation of blood to the head and brain.

A gentleman then had a rather unusual query in that, when he awoke in the morning, his eyes were completely closed and he could only open them with great difficulty. He asked Dr Vogel for some advice as to what he thought could be wrong. He said he had no discharge but Vogel and I agreed that he certainly had conjunctivitis, which can take a long time to clear. Vogel suggested he tried the old-fashioned remedy of chamomile compresses, which could be of tremendous help in such circumstances.

Another lively discussion then developed when a young lady said that it was not unusual for her not to go to the toilet for ten days. Although she was not unduly worried about this, Vogel was. He said that constipation can have several causes but when the large intestine is subject to metabolic changes then this can indicate a serious problem and everything possible must be done to alleviate the situation. The first thing he asked her to do was to study her diet, starting with what she ate for breakfast – which, in her case, was appalling. He recommended she eat muesli with the addition of some cooked prunes and prune juice, and to add to this a teaspoonful of *Linoforce*. This effective remedy offers relief by combining the gentle bulking action of linseed with the stimulating effects of senna leaves. As I mentioned in a previous chapter, if you do not export in 24 hours what you have consumed during that same period, then you are encouraging problems. Time must be taken to chew food thoroughly and, as Vogel said, your best digestive aid is saliva. Never postpone going to the toilet. Drink at least two glasses of lukewarm water first thing in the morning and make sure that you take plenty of exercise (whether it be in the form of walking, swimming or cycling). If the problem persists, then you should consult your doctor.

Vogel also commented that having a normal motion every day would have a beneficial effect on her weight and, as she had problems controlling her weight, she was pleased to hear that positive information.

Next followed a question from a lady in her 60s who suffered from daily nosebleeds. She said it was impossible for her to stop the bleeding and, although she had been to the doctor, she was still having problems, often at the most inopportune moments. Vogel believed that her blood vessels were weak but suggested a useful technique would be to press firmly on the relevant part of her nose until the bleeding stopped. If that failed, then she could take the rather bizarre step of placing a piece of fresh chicken meat up the appropriate nostril and then the bleeding would stop immediately. However, he said, a much simpler way would be to take *Bursa pastoris* tincture, which often proves to be most effective. This particular woman said she would try anything to stop this problem – even if it meant going into her fridge for a piece of fresh chicken meat!

Another woman said she was becoming forgetful and asked if anything could be done to improve this worrying situation. I was pleased that Vogel recalled the time we spent in Korea, as he told her about an elderly man there who chewed *Ginkgo biloba* leaves every day to keep his mind alert. As Vogel said, it is vital that the brain remains active. He asked her to ensure that she had ample relaxation and plenty of exercise, and also stressed the importance of keeping an eye on her cholesterol levels. He pointed out that a cholesterol level above 5.2 was not acceptable and that a lot of avoidable problems could develop if she didn't keep an eye on that. To lower cholesterol levels he recommended porridge in the morning, chewing the seeds from grapes, taking some *Milk Thistle Complex* and eating plenty of garlic.

This led to an elderly lady asking if anything could be done to combat osteoporosis. Vogel explained that a loss in bone mass can be experienced from the age of 40 onwards. There can be many causes, for example drinking too much alcohol, smoking, or having too much salt, animal protein, coffee, tea or chocolate in the diet. Vogel strongly advised people with osteoporosis to take the homoeopathic preparation *Urticalcin*, which I discussed earlier. If taken daily, it provides extra help in maintaining strong bones.

Another listener asked about hay fever. Vogel informed him that cases of hay fever were increasing annually, due in large part to the widespread growth of rapeseed. Those who suffer from hay fever should also be aware that they run the risk of developing arthritis or rheumatism. The first thing to do is look at the patient's diet and reduce their intake of milk, cheese and salt. It would also be of great benefit for them to start taking the remedy *Luffa Complex* from the end of March until the hay fever season is over. If one knows a good homoeopathic doctor, then an injection of a homoeopathic remedy can be given before the season starts but, as I have said, one of the finest things to take is *Luffa Complex*. From extensive research into this excellent product, it has also been shown to be helpful to those who are allergic to dust mites.

A tremendous range of questions were asked that evening. Another listener asked what could be done to ease the pain from wasp stings. Wasp stings can be very dangerous if the person who is stung is allergic to them. They can develop anaphylactic shock, displaying difficulty in breathing, swelling in the throat, itching or fainting. If someone exhibits any of these symptoms, it is imperative that they are taken to hospital straight away, as this condition can be fatal. In less serious cases, where the symptoms are swelling and discomfort, the quickest way to alleviate this is to take five drops of *Apis D4* straight away and repeat a further two times a day. Great relief can also be achieved by dabbing some tea tree oil onto the sting. But, above all, try and keep away from wasps! Citronella oil or *Po-Ho Oil* are good deterrents for bees, wasps and midges.

Another question was from a young girl who had tremendous problems with halitosis – in other words, bad breath. She told Vogel that she made sure that her teeth and gums were very healthy and she took great care with oral hygiene but, nevertheless, her boyfriend wanted to end their relationship because he found the situation repellent.

Many people suffer from this problem and Vogel told her that the most common cause is a disturbance in the bowel bacteria. He advised her to eliminate white sugar and white flour from her diet, to chew her food thoroughly, to keep her consumption of milk and cheese to a minimum and to take a teaspoonful of

Molkosan twice daily, together with 20 drops of *Milk Thistle Complex*, also twice a day. He reassured her that, by making these changes to her diet, she would see a definite improvement. I would add that it would also be a good idea to take 15 drops of *Peppermint Complex* twice a day and to take 3 garlic capsules last thing at night, as this is an excellent deodoriser.

A man then put up his hand and pleaded with Dr Vogel to help him because he had to rise five times during the night to go to the toilet. As he said, 'When I have to go, I have to go.' He explained that he had been to see a urologist and was told he had prostate problems but, because of his advancing years, he felt it unwise to undergo an operation. Vogel answered him by saying that if help is sought quickly, then prostate problems can be easily treated. If left untreated for a long time, however, the situation becomes more difficult. He recommended the man take a handful of pumpkin seeds every day, together with some *Saw Palmetto Complex* (previously known as *Prostasan*), which, he assured him, would help a lot. He also said to make sure that he took enough exercise and kept his body moving, by walking, swimming or cycling, and emphasised the importance of keeping constipation at bay. He also urged him to keep a careful eye on such culprits as herbs, strong spices (like chilli), coffee and alcohol, and to restrict his intake of fluids after 6 p.m. Additional relief could also be achieved by rubbing *St John's Wort Oil* over the bladder area and between the legs.

That particular lecture proved to be such a success, with many people leaving much wiser than when they arrived. From the various questions that were asked, I too gained a lot of practical wisdom, which I have put to good use in helping people with their different ailments throughout the world.

Chapter 12

Man has not one body but three – a physical, a mental and an emotional body.

Jan de Vries

In the eighteenth century, a man called Samuel Hahnemann travelled all the way from his homeland of Germany to visit the oldest medical school in Europe, which is now part of Edinburgh University. Hahnemann is credited with being the founder of homoeopathy as we know it today and while in Edinburgh he had a lively conversation with his peer, Professor Merridge. When the professor asked him, 'What is health?' Dr Hahnemann immediately fired back at him, 'What is illness?' Basically, illness is disharmony wherever it surfaces in the body, 'an aberration from the state of health' – whether physical, mental or emotional.

Vogel subscribed to many of Hahnemann's beliefs. He too was conscious of the fact that in order to achieve the best result for patients, it was not solely a matter of treating the physical symptoms; the mental and emotional state of a patient also had to be taken into account in order to harmonise the entire body. As I learned while I was studying in China, this principle is also fundamental to Chinese medicine, especially acupuncture – the aim of which is to harmonise that which is out of harmony in the body. The importance which the Chinese have long attributed to this state of being becomes gloriously apparent when you visit the Forbidden City in Beijing. One of the most amazing rooms in this breathtaking complex is the hall of Supreme Harmony, which was used for important state occasions such as the enthronement of the Crown Prince, the celebration of the Emperor's birthday, and so on.

Today, many serious health problems are resulting from a lack of harmony in people's bodies and their lives in general. Sadly, problems caused by emotional imbalance are increasing at an alarming rate as people's mental health is under sustained attack in the modern world, with the result that more and more people are seeking relief through strong pharmaceutical products that can be very addictive. The side effects of drugs such as tranquillisers and anti-depressants have received a lot of attention in the media in recent years, and of course these drugs only treat the symptoms of the problem rather than getting down to the root cause. It is very important when treating patients that we achieve harmony between the three bodies, and this is where complementary medicine, with its use of herbal or homoeopathic remedies, is of great benefit.

Over the course of his research, Hahnemann developed four fundamental principles. The first of these is '*similia similibus curentur*' or 'like cures like'. This means that a remedy that produces symptoms of a disease when given to a healthy patient can alleviate the problem in a patient suffering from the disease. This discovery can be applied to any condition and to any individual – in measles, for instance, the principle is not to suppress the illness, but to bring it out of the body. A homoeopathic remedy will probably make the measles a little worse before they are out of the system. Instead of assuming that symptoms represent illogical, improper or unhealthy responses that should be treated with drugs or surgery, Hahnemann believed that symptoms are positive, adaptive responses of the body to deal with an imbalance that has occurred. It is often said that God's creation, the body, is very intelligent – in fact, supremely intelligent.

The second principle is 'the minimum dose', which resulted from Hahnemann's attempts to work out a way of administering therapeutic doses of medicines while avoiding side effects. He believed that large doses of drugs actually made a patient's condition worse, while small, diluted doses enabled the body to fight off the disease. The way that he produced medicines was called 'potentiation' – the third principle. Homoeopathic remedies are made through a process of serial dilution, and the remedy is vigorously shaken through each stage to ensure its dynamic nature. Finally, the fourth principle is 'the single remedy', meaning that only one homoeopathic remedy should be administered at a time.

Homoeopathic practitioners believe that people differ in the way their bodies react to an illness, according to their temperament. Consequently, this calls for the need to match the characteristics of the patient (i.e. taking into consideration their temperament, personality and emotional and physical states) with the remedy to be prescribed (whether it be a plant, mineral or other substance). A homoeopath therefore studies the person as a whole, treating the individual rather than just the disease. As a result, patients suffering from the same illness may actually be prescribed different remedies, which many people find difficult to comprehend.

Vogel and I were certain that God had created a remedy in nature to treat every illness and disease but believed that it is up to man to find the particular remedy that should be administered. It is, therefore, vital that the practitioner treating the patient is educated in the ways of homoeopathy, because one incorrectly prescribed remedy – even in its lowest potency – can cause a great deal of damage. Throughout our many years of practice, both Vogel and I unfortunately came across many cases where such damage had been done by wrongly prescribed medicines. One woman who stands out in my mind came to see me while I was giving a talk in a health food store in Kent. She had been suffering with various problems for over two years and told me that she had been prescribed the constitutional remedy *Sepia*. While this can be a wonderful remedy and has helped many people, it was completely unsuitable for this woman's symptoms, which had continued to get worse. I immediately prescribed *Ovarium* and she soon contacted me to thank me, as she was feeling so much better.

I cannot praise Vogel enough for the extensive research he carried out – even to the extent of testing remedies on himself – before prescribing a product. He went to great lengths to ensure that his remedies had no side effects and, as part of this process, he considered the effects that the treatments would have on all three bodies of Man. As described earlier, these brilliant remedies have provided the backbone for my work throughout the world.

Vogel and I talked a lot about Hahnemann's methods, one of which was to form an image of a person – and by looking at that image and talking to the patient, it becomes easier to determine where the problem may lie. I recall a mother and her little girl who came to talk to us following one particular lecture. I immediately sensed which type of characteristics this child had and realised that she was very much what we would term a '*Pulsatilla* child'. The person usually in need of *Pulsatilla* is a blue-eyed, blonde-haired individual, has a sensitive disposition, bursts into tears easily, needs comfort, hates quarrelling, has difficulty in digesting fatty foods, sometimes has poor circulation and, because the *Pulsatilla* type is often over-conscientious, has problems with the ears, bladder infections and diarrhoea. When answering Vogel's questions, the mother confirmed that these were precisely the problems affecting her child, who particularly suffered from recurrent bladder infections. Vogel and I had come to the same conclusion about this child without exchanging a single word. As her whole constitution pointed to the fact that she really needed to be treated as a *Pulsatilla* child, I wrote down on a piece of paper that her mother should give her *Pulsatilla D6*. A very grateful letter later followed from her, stating that, within a week, her daughter's problems had cleared up.

In homoeopathy, the combination of an individual's physical and mental characteristics is called their 'constitution', and *Pulsatilla* is what would be described as a constitutional remedy. When such a remedy is applied, one has to be extremely careful, as sometimes the symptoms will initially get worse. This is because, as Hahnemann advocated, there is a requirement to stimulate the body's own defence mechanisms to fight the illness and remove it from the body rather than, as in conventional medicine, suppressing the symptoms and, thus, keeping the illness within the body.

As was stressed to this child's mother, it is important when a constitutional remedy is prescribed that the patient gets plenty of fresh air, lots of rest and is kept warm. With the older *Pulsatilla* types, we often come across additional ailments such as headaches and menstrual problems.

This brings to mind another case that Vogel and I worked on together, where we had confirmation of Hahnemann's principles being so appropriate in this day and age. In this instance, we were consulted by a young policeman's wife. She was totally despondent when she first came to see us. Not only had she been on the verge of ending her own life on several occasions but she had also almost ended the lives of her husband and two children when she lost control and tried to drive her car into the river in an attempt to drown them. Various specialists had diagnosed her condition completely incorrectly – with their opinions varying from depression to ME – and some even admitted that they did not know what was wrong with her. When we saw her, however, I quickly remarked to Vogel that she had many characteristics of someone in need of *Gentiana*.

After finding out a bit about her medical history, Vogel and I were in total agreement that she had serious problems. Her lymph glands in her neck, armpits and groin were all swollen – and I commented to Vogel that her whole system seemed to be poisoned. Our diagnosis was confirmed when the results of a blood test showed high levels of toxicity within her body. Her lymph system had become completely congested with waste material, which had infected her blood and, as a result, her system had become very toxic. She had a lot of amalgam in the fillings in her teeth, her diet was appalling and, due to her prolonged ill health, a great strain had been put on her relationship with her husband.

We both looked at this woman who was so poorly and distraught. She was physically, mentally and emotionally imbalanced. I suggested that we started by giving her a combination of *Gentiana* and the homoeopathic remedy called *Arsenicum*, and then carry out a thorough detoxification. We started to treat her with the two constitutional remedies – one to be taken for the first month, then followed by the second – talked to her at length about ways of improving her diet and, following that, detoxified her system with the *Detox Box* of Dr Vogel. This is a ten-day elimination programme during which the patient takes *Calendula Complex*, *Frangula Complex*, *Milk Thistle Complex* and *Solidago Complex* in regulated amounts.

As her immune system had been given a tremendous knock, it took us some time before we were able to make a breakthrough but eventually she made a steady recovery and has never looked back.

The Vogel *Detox Box* arose from a discussion that Alfred and I had during a trip to Canada in the 1970s. One morning while we were eating breakfast in the hotel restaurant, we looked around at the variety of different foods people were eating. When we noticed what one particular family had selected, we both shook our heads. Because I practise Chinese facial diagnosis, I commented to Vogel that the entire family had liver toxicity. We then discussed the best way in which to give the body a thorough spring clean. As a consequence of that talk, the *Detox Box* was conceived, which is now recognised all over the world as being one of the finest products on the market. Detoxification is not only a great way of spring cleaning the gall bladder, liver, bowel, kidneys and stomach, but it also starts the detoxification process of the lymph system.

During a later trip to San Francisco, when I conducted a consultation in a health food store, I learned that this treatment was particularly popular there because in that part of the United States there was a lot of pollution in the air and people wanted to do everything they could to clear it from their system. Later on, I devised a diet to be used in conjunction with the *Detox Box* and, today, I am happy to see that this treatment is still sold all over the world.

To find harmony between the physical, mental and emotional bodies is not an easy task. We have to contend with a lot of negative influences such as pollution, which undoubtedly has played an enormous role in the escalation of many modern illnesses and diseases. Now in the twenty-first century, we are witnessing a daily increase in the number of people suffering from allergies, as their immune systems are unable to cope with the poisonous chemicals that are all around us. As well as pollution, allergic reactions can be caused by such things as artificial food colourings, but whatever the cause they should be seen as an alarm bell indicating that something in the body needs attention. This situation is only made worse by the increase in stress caused by pressures at work, unforeseen circumstances and unhappiness. Health problems resulting from asthma and bronchitis are also increasing by the day.

I remember when a girl, aged about eight, came to see us. She was in complete turmoil. Not only did she suffer from hyperventilation and panic attacks but she was also slightly asthmatic. When we started to dig into her medical history, we soon discovered where her problems lay. Her system was being attacked by three obvious problems, namely, (a) her living conditions, (b) her unhappy family life, and (c) the most appalling diet. That unfortunate child was taking three different inhalers, in addition to other medication, just to keep her condition under control. The house in which she lived was filthy, exacerbating her allergy to dust, and her life circumstances in general were appalling.

In an attempt to get her condition under control, we first looked at ways of improving her diet, which entailed the withdrawal of cow's milk and cheese, and the introduction of supplements of B, C, D and E vitamins. We prescribed the anti-allergy homoeopathic remedy *Luffa Complex*, which is also ideal for desensitising the system, together with herbal *Drosinula Syrup* and some *Passiflora* to make her calmer. I also taught her some exercises to help her relax and gave her some acupuncture. Importantly, I was also able to talk to her parents about the home situation and gave them advice about diet and lifestyle. Later on, I also added some homoeopathic remedies to her treatment. She was a lovely girl, who thankfully followed our advice to the letter. Today, when I still sometimes see her, I think back to what her circumstances once were. Her case is a perfect example of how it is important not just to treat a patient's physical symptoms but also to look beyond these and get to the root of the problem as best we can.

I am aware that we all lead busy lives today, but it is now more important than ever that we make time to look thoroughly into the background of illnesses and diseases to try and find out how they started and in what circumstances they developed. This reminds me of a young woman who came to see me while Vogel was working with me in Scotland. Although this girl consulted us about a minor problem, we both became aware that, deep down, there was more to it than she had led us to believe. It was only when we examined her situation in greater detail that we both became aware that she was suicidal. She finally confided in us that she had personal problems – and this is where homoeopathy often comes into its own. When we carefully delved a bit deeper into her background, we realised that she was actually suffering from a severe emotional imbalance. It emerged that she had been in a relationship for many years but the relationship never really progressed and, when she finally realised that her boyfriend had been stringing her along, she became extremely distressed, as she was very fond of him. Sadly, women often take relationships far more seriously than men and it is easy to appreciate how such an emotional incident can have a detrimental effect on a person, like this girl, who was actually slowly dying of a broken heart. This might sound implausible but I have actually witnessed this happening once during the years I have been in practice.

When we chatted a little bit more to her, and Vogel and I pointed out certain things to her, sharing with her a few things we had learned about life and relationships along the way, she nodded, and I could see that she was starting to take in what we were saying and beginning to trust us. It became apparent that she was also consumed with jealousy, as this particular fellow had been seeing other women while involved with her but, even in spite of this, she still loved him so much.

We realised we had our work cut out in getting this emotional upset completely out of her system but, thankfully, we were eventually able to help her. In addition to some homoeopathic remedies, we also prescribed some flower remedies and after she had recovered from this whole unpleasant experience, she asked me to explain how we had been able to treat her. I told her that the symptoms she had were not the disease, only evidence of a disease, and that one of the benefits of homoeopathy is that it goes to the source of the problem. I told this young lady that she had been completely out of tune with her body because of her failed relationship and, as mentioned earlier, the three bodies (mental, emotional and physical) must be in tune with each other to bring harmony. The constitutional remedy that we used in this instance was *Aurum* and she listened intently as I told her that, in homoeopathy, we have learned the precision of a healing system which conceives all symptoms as part of a larger whole, which appears to stimulate the body's natural force, rather than attacking parts. Homoeopathy will work with us, not against us.

Unfortunately, many people are still sceptical about homoeopathy. I remember once taking part in a radio programme in Dublin with the Irish broadcaster Pat Kenny when a doctor phoned in to condemn homoeopathy, saying that it was quackery and the results had never been proven. I told him that, on the contrary, a group of medical students in Utrecht had researched this very subject for more than ten years and had proved that even the lowest potency of a homoeopathic remedy affected the production of saliva, indicating that it effected change in the body.

I remember when I was invited to attend an important talk given for health insurers in Holland. As the main speaker was one of the most eminent pharmacologists in Holland, this generated a lot of interest, which was evident by the number of professors, doctors and scientists who attended. I wasn't terribly pleased at having to be present at that particular talk as I felt this professor was opposed to homoeopathy and herbal medicine. This was confirmed when he started the discussion by saying that the benefits of homoeopathy could be likened to the situation where a little boy fell in the street and his mother gently kissed his wound to make it better – it offered comfort but not real results.

A very lively debate developed and at the end he admitted that I had managed to make him think again. Not long after that particular discussion, which was covered extensively in the Dutch media, Vogel had an interview with that particular professor. I was very interested when the professor told him that most doctors in Holland were major users of herbal remedies. Vogel told him that even in countries where the governments were opposed to natural medicine, herbal medicine was taking over, as people wanted freedom of choice. As Vogel and I often said, you cannot argue with results.

There is a growing consensus in the world that the massive amount of money allocated to medical research has failed to achieve any significant improvement in Western societies' levels of health. The incidence of major, chronic diseases like cancer, diabetes and heart disease continue to climb, and homoeopathy offers a time-tested method that meets the need for additional non-toxic therapy. It is reassuring to know that, when homoeopathic remedies are administered properly, there are no side effects. This is a very important part of the whole concept of homoeopathy, which encompasses all areas of medical care, from prevention to emergency and acute care, as well as the treatment of chronic diseases. It offers the individual improved health and quality of life. As I stated in my previous book, *Fifty Years Fighting*, I cannot understand why medical practitioners would resist this system, or why they would insist on administering aggressive drugs instead of looking for a more natural solution.

Luckily a change of attitude is now taking place all over the world with more and more scientific tests being carried out to prove the efficacy of herbal and homoeopathic remedies. As we are gaining ground, it is greatly encouraging to see how natural medicine works in instances where orthodox remedies might have failed. I often mention one of Vogel's sayings in lectures, 'We are born in nature, we belong to nature and if we obey the laws of nature, then we obey the laws of God.'

Chapter 13

It is very important to be in tune with your body.
Jan de Vries

Nowadays, many people in the Western world are obsessed with body image. It would, however, be more beneficial if they became familiar with the way their body works rather than just the way it looks, as it is vital that we learn to recognise the warning signs when something may be going wrong. The last thing I want to do is turn people into hypochondriacs or neurotics but we need to pay attention to our bodies when they tell us to 'STOP'. A lot of people, including myself, often ignore the warning signs and try to carry on regardless. If this is allowed to happen, then the body will draw on its own reserve energies, and as soon as these energies become low, our immune system is laid open to attack. This is what happened to me in Australia when I contracted a virus and then developed diabetes. I had been working too hard, preparing for Alfred's arrival, and my resistance to infection was low.

Contrary to general opinion, you cannot catch a virus easily; the body must be susceptible to attack, and this can have disastrous results.

It is most annoying if we hear a few notes at a concert that are out of tune. We then say, 'That is not right.' I wish it was possible to deal with the body's imbalances as easily as we can deal with an out-of-tune musical instrument.

The other day, I had a visit from a lady who was 103. It was apparent that she was incredibly alert and intelligent from the questions she asked me and she also told me about the daily duties she was still able to attend to. I was so impressed at how sharp-witted she was that I knew there must be an explanation, so I explained to her that I was in the process of gathering a wide variety of information for a new series of books that I was going to write called *Jan de Vries' Health Secrets*. I told her a little about my great friend Alfred Vogel, remarking on how fresh his mind had been right up to the end and how he had given me many tips, and then I asked her if she would mind letting me into her own secret. She told me the same thing that my grandmother had told me when she was 98 years of age: 'The secret to good health and a bright mind is to keep yourself up to date with everything.' Although by that time in her life my grandmother could no longer see and needed the help of an assistant, she still made sure that she kept her mind active by doing daily crosswords.

This lady told me that as well as keeping up to date she kept in tune with her body and whenever something went wrong – even if it was something like a minor cold – she took action straight away. She is one of the countless people who believes that *Echinaforce* from Dr Vogel is an outstanding remedy and, like Vogel (who used *Echinaforce* throughout his life because of the fine composition of this remedy), she didn't believe in discontinuing it. She informed me that she had been taking *Echinaforce* for the last 30 years, 'to keep me fit and healthy'. I am often asked if there is any reason why *Echinaforce* cannot be taken continuously and my view is that *Echinacea* is an immune booster while *Echinaforce* is an immune balancer. *Echinacea* should be taken when immunity may be low to give the system a boost, while *Echinaforce* helps to maintain a high level of immunity. During the 50 years I have been in practice and in all the years I have worked with *Echinaforce*, I can honestly say that I have never come across a single side effect and I have witnessed the tremendous benefits that people have obtained from this excellent treatment.

This elderly lady was very well informed, as she told me that she had read about Samuel Hahnemann's belief in the vital force in the body and wanted to ask me about it. He said something along the lines of, 'I make sure that my vital organs are taken care of and that the vital force is in tune.' It is this vital force and its healing mechanism which are stimulated by homoeopathic or herbal remedies, and naturopathic therapy is used to release blockages which sometimes can occur in this vital force. Hahnemann put a lot of emphasis on the fact that the vital force should flow freely. In my own practice, I have often seen in acupuncture that, by relieving one small energy blockage, the whole body is then allowed to strive to get back into tune.

We see with homoeopathic remedies that they often work as an adjunctive and supportive mechanism to standard medical therapies. They are certainly not a replacement. The medical establishment, however, sometimes believe that this is the aim of complementary therapists – to replace them – and there are those who would like to see homoeopathy banned for that reason. Although this medical art has been used for centuries to treat illness, it was not designed for severe or chronic conditions, and we really have to try and understand how they work. My 103-year-old patient was completely familiar with that fact and I was amazed how, even with some of the constitutional remedies that she told me about, she was able to control some pain that she experienced.

It is quite amazing what one is capable of achieving with the use of homoeopathic remedies. This lady mentioned to me how she once managed to clear a nasty allergy by taking Vogel's *Luffa Complex*, and as I had a little time to spare, I told her the story about the development of this remedy, in which she was totally engrossed.

I am still acquainted with the Swiss chemist who had a tremendous input into Vogel's remedies. He worked on *Luffa Complex* with his team of co-workers and they developed this marvellous preparation by combining seven healthy plants from various parts of the world, though, of course, Vogel was involved at every stage. The first ingredient used was *Cardiospermum halicacabum*, which was later discovered to be extremely valuable in the treatment of allergies and skin problems, and is found in large quantities in Madeira. It also contains a North African remedy called *Ammi visnaga* (or *Khella*) which comes from the bark of a tree and is used to bring relief to those suffering from cramps and spasms. In addition, it contains a natural histamine which makes it invaluable to hay fever sufferers. *Oukababa* is another component, which is taken from the bark of a tree in West Africa and is regularly used to neutralise poisons. *Aralia racemosa* comes from North America and is of remarkable help in treating respiratory problems and troublesome coughs. Mexico is the source of the next two ingredients. A plant called *Galphimia glauca* grows there, which greatly helps strengthen the tissues in the body, while the *Creasotum* plant, which has quite a pleasant scent, can be found in the north of the country. Finally, there is *Luffa Operculata*, one of the main ingredients in *Luffa Complex*. This comes from Columbia. So, natural resources from around the world have been brought together to formulate this excellent remedy, which I have often prescribed with great success for those whose bodies are slightly out of tune.

While writing this chapter, I recalled an elegant, young couple who came to see me one busy Saturday. They made such an attractive pair and, yet, I could see by the expressions on their faces that something was bothering them. They were certainly in tune with each other, but their body energies were completely out of tune. It does not take a lot for this to happen and everyday incidents can easily accelerate this imbalance. The man was almost in tears as he told me that everything had been fine until one day when he was at work he got a phone call to inform him that his mother had died that afternoon. The person who conveyed this message was certainly not diplomatic and this news had a devastating impact on the fellow. The following day, he felt unwell and started to cough (which was probably a nervous cough). With each day that passed, he became more ill, and his wife became worried when she realised that he was still not right after his mother's funeral.

A series of little incidents occurred which caused his health to go completely out of tune. Unfortunately, he didn't want to communicate with anyone and had become totally withdrawn. On top of that, his sexual desires had diminished to such a level that he no longer felt capable of having a loving relationship with his wife. He was a sad young man but, as he said, he had an attractive wife who showed him great compassion and they would do anything possible to get things back in order.

There were a lot of things that needed to be done. First, he still had not come to terms with the grief he felt for his late mother and, to offer him some help in this direction, I prescribed *Ignatia*, which greatly assists in taking the sting out of bereavement. He had an extremely unhealthy diet and had started to drink excessively as a way of drowning his sorrows, which, of course, had the effect of further reducing his sexual appetite and he felt he had come to the end of the road. I went over all this with him in detail, then adjusted his diet and, because he was desperate to get well, he was very willing to cooperate. I introduced wheatgerm into his diet and even included some wheatgerm capsules from Dr Vogel. I managed to cleanse his liver with the introduction of *Milk Thistle Complex* and then stimulated his prostate (as he also had problems in that area) with the fresh herbal extract *Saw Palmetto*. I also prescribed some *Vitality Essence*, together with some extra Vogel vitamins. He reported to me three weeks later that things were starting to improve, except he still had many problems with his sleep pattern. We managed to rectify this with some *Valerian Hops* (25 drops taken half an hour before going to bed).

Surprisingly, within a very short space of time, he was back in tune with his body. This, in turn, made him see things more positively and he was able to appreciate his wife again. I saw them some time later while still writing this book and they reminded me of the importance of being in tune with your body.

Chapter 14

Nature always overrules science.

Jan de Vries

A middle-aged lady came to see me at my London clinic the other day looking extremely healthy and happy. Although she is now living abroad and I had not seen her for a number of years, I instantly recognised her. Her friendly smile now lit up her face but I could not help but remember a very different picture, as we had experienced an particularly anxious time when trying to treat her as a young girl. She smiled at me as she said, 'Can you believe how well I am? I now have three children, and I just wanted to come to tell you how grateful I am for everything you have done for me.'

I was so pleased to see her because I sometimes get depressed when I dwell on the many illnesses and diseases I see every day. It is very heartening when one is able to see the evidence of how nature can help people, particularly those who have come to the end of the road in terms of what conventional medicine can offer them. This particular patient had been crippled with arthritis at a very young age. Her doctors were unable to help her but, thankfully, with the application of acupuncture and the prescription of some remedies, I was able to turn her situation around.

I was once called to a London hospital where I found the distraught parents of a young girl sitting helplessly at her bedside. They had come from Nigeria in the hope of finding help but the doctors were baffled as to what was wrong with their daughter until they eventually diagnosed systemic lupus erythematosus (SLE). This is a chronic, multi-system inflammatory disease that can affect any and every organ, and by the time the diagnosis was made, she was in such a bad way that she was not expected to live more than a few weeks.

From her bed, the young girl looked up at me with big brown eyes as if pleading, 'Please help me.' I talked to her and, indeed, I too was worried because, after carrying out some iris diagnosis, feeling her pulse and looking at her tongue, I could see that her system was being poisoned. She had an extremely congested lymphatic system and a lot of skin problems, both of which are indicators of SLE. I took a blood sample, which was extensively researched and, from that, it was concluded that a lot of poisonous material had been accumulating in her system, probably for a few years.

I immediately set about prescribing some remedies for her – such as a strong antioxidant, *Petasites*, very high levels of vitamin C and as much beetroot juice as she could drink. After I saw the results of her blood test, I also phoned Alfred Vogel and explained the situation to him. As luck would have it, he said that he was actually going to be taking a break from his travels to visit London and he would be willing to see her.

A week later, he joined me at the bedside of this young girl in one of London's foremost hospitals. Vogel was also shocked at what he saw and said that we would need to use a strange, old-fashioned remedy that his grandmother regularly used when faced with serious problems. I was fascinated by his story of how the roots of couch grass were extremely helpful in cases such as this and immediately went to get some fresh couch grass juice via a friend in London who had agreed to help us. Vogel looked at her compassionately, took her pulse and said, 'I am sure she is going to make it.' Although she was critically ill at that time, he was right.

As soon as she awakened each morning, this young girl was given a small glass of fresh couch grass juice to drink. Fortunately I had planned to be in London for a few days and was therefore able to call on her after she had taken the initial dose. As her temperature continued to rise, the doctors were becoming increasingly alarmed that she would not pull through but, nevertheless, they were all willing to help. Once she started to show signs of improvement, they began to have faith in what we were doing and became so supportive that they left it up to us to do what we felt necessary as, scientifically, they could do nothing further to help this young girl. The end result was that she survived – with a simple helping hand from nature.

I have experienced many times in practice that nature can overrule science. Often it is not until we give nature a chance that we discover the solution to a problem.

I have told the story many times of when I was in a quandary over a patient's needs and Vogel advised me to go to the seaside or into the fields to ponder over what nature could offer to help. I am pleased to say that I have never been disappointed by the many answers that have sometimes been literally lying at my feet. The answer often becomes clear when I can actually see the herbs, plants or even trees which might offer me a clue, through their signatures or characteristics, as to what I should use to help a patient.

Situated across from Vogel's house was the Ida Wegmann Institute and I vividly recollect when we went there to study what they were practising. Vogel reminded me of one of their main remedies – *Mistletoe* (*Viscum album*) – and explained why they had chosen mistletoe preparations to help treat cancer patients. When he saw mistletoe growing in an oak tree, he used to say to me, 'Look what that is doing. The mistletoe is growing like a parasite on the tree just as cancer grows like a parasite in the human body.' It has been proved that *Mistletoe* can stimulate cell metabolism and, as this is generally weak in cancer patients, mistletoe preparations offer a valuable treatment. It is sometimes known as 'the plant of life and death', as it has both negatives and positives. It gives a clear message – 'Please use me. I am growing here like a parasite, killing this tree, just as cancer does, in this tree of life, which is what Man really is. Use me homoeopathically so that I can attack and kill off the cancer cells in the body, which are slowly killing this life within us.' During my years in practice, I have repeatedly been amazed at the remarkable results that can be achieved by using this parasitic plant.

Sometimes we are blind to what is going on around us. We must open our eyes to find the herb, plant or tree created by God that can help us. I am a firm believer that God has kept his promise by supplying us with everything in nature that we need to heal and protect our health – although it is up to Man to discover how these plants can be used. Instead of spending millions of pounds in finding out what happens on the moon or in examining the stars, we should be investigating and researching what is out there in nature and how it can be used to alleviate human suffering. After all, that is our greatest responsibility. Vogel used to say in his lectures, 'We are each other's debtors. We have to help each other in this often difficult life, and by sharing in each other's difficulties, we are helping wherever we can, which is of the utmost importance.'

A well-known gentleman entered my consulting room recently. I immediately recognised him and was aware of the high position he held. He looked sharply at me and, before even sitting down, asked, 'Do you practise intuitive medicine?' As nobody had ever asked me that before, I pondered over it for a moment. I asked him to sit down and enquired what he really meant by his question. He explained that he had followed my work for a long time, had read my books and was of the opinion that I must do a lot through intuition. He then asked if I believed in the sixth sense. I replied that I believed there are five tangible senses and, indeed, I did believe that intuition was a sixth sense. This response seemed to reassure him, as he then said he wanted me to treat him. I proceeded to examine him, carried out the necessary tests to confirm what was wrong and, fortunately, his treatment was successful.

Whilst writing this book, and thinking about that particular gentleman, I recalled an incident that took place an extremely long time ago when Alfred Vogel and I were waiting for the arrival of our train. A young family of five were also at the station – the parents and their three children. In that dank station, Vogel focused his attention on one particular child and became eager to talk to the family. Eventually he went up to them and enquired what was wrong with their child. The mother started to cry and said she was so pleased that we had approached them, even though she had no idea who Vogel or I were. With Vogel's knowledge and experience, he intuitively knew that there was something seriously wrong with that child and he wanted the mother's confirmation that he was correct. As it turned out, the parents stated that their daughter had leukaemia.

While Vogel spoke to these parents, he asked me to take down some notes. He then explained who he was and offered his help. He asked me to send some medicines for this child, free of charge. He assured the family that we would keep in contact with them and help their child to the best of our ability. After we had all the information we needed about this young girl, and received her parents' agreement to treat her, their train arrived and, as it pulled out of the station, I caught a glimpse of the happy expression on Vogel's face as he had yet again given help where it was needed. Many years have passed since our encounter at that dark station when everyone showed concern for that lovely young girl. Her parents wrote faithfully to me and, today, it is comforting to know that their daughter is alive and well.

There are often outward signs of what is happening inwardly. It was for that reason that I studied Chinese facial diagnosis and also the type of outgoing energy each individual possesses. Scientifically, that can be difficult to explain, but when one is close to nature, one often finds the answers.

Vogel was also blessed with a seventh sense. When he was faced with tremendous worries, he tried to look at problems from a humorous angle. That seventh sense – the sense of humour – was something that frequently helped him through difficult times. Like Vogel, having a sense of humour has helped me when things have not been easy, as I have written in the second part of my autobiography, *Fifty Years Fighting*. It is therefore important to look forward and never to lose that sense of humour. After all, it takes much less effort to smile than to frown.

When I helped to launch Vogel's first book in Holland, *The Nature Doctor*, I was very aware that he had written it as he wanted to share his knowledge with others. It soon sold over 500,000 copies. Virtually every household in Holland now owns a copy and it has sold over 2,500,000 worldwide. This book, however, is only the tip of the iceberg in relation to the knowledge Vogel had. It provides first-hand advice on natural healing methods but he ends this informative book by saying:

> On the other hand, let me say that there is one little 'herb' I do not know either, the one referred to in an old proverb: 'There's many a herb to cure, Not one, however, for death, to be sure.' I am fully aware that my medical advice is but a help for dealing with the times in which we live.

We only have one chance at this life and so we must make the most of it. No one wants to live with problems, so we must do all we can to minimise or eliminate difficulties. On a daily basis in my practice I hear patients say, 'Oh well, I have a problem. I will have to live with it.' This is not true. If you have a problem, then you must make every effort to eradicate it, in order to have as fulfilling a life as possible.

It is said that 'you get out of life what you put into it', or 'you reap what you sow'. When we invest in our health, it is essential that we do so sensibly. As I have said in a previous chapter, there is nothing common about common sense. We should all set aside some time to sit down and contemplate where we are going wrong. Our own intuition will guide us and help us to restore balance. If we have lost that sense, then we have lost everything. My mother used to stress the importance of listening 'to your inner voice', which will tell us what we should or shouldn't do. By being in tune with our bodies, we will achieve greater happiness and enjoy good health.

In coming to the end of this autobiography, I would like to add how grateful I am to my Creator for letting me be a little part in this life. Although I am only a small drop in the ocean, it is comforting to know that everyone on earth belongs to that ocean. I am also grateful to those who have shown me the way to truth, reality and understanding. When I look at the sun, the moon and stars, the fields, the trees and flowers – in fact, all that is around us – I am thankful that I am a small part of that great creation, where I have seen that nature will always overrule science.

Although we live in a world of great unrest, terrorism and unhappiness, we have to look forward to the future that lies before us, to a time when we will be able to conquer illness and untimely death.

The last time I met with my great friend Alfred Vogel, we reflected, with grateful thanks, on the many years we had worked together and the part we had been able to play in alleviating human suffering. Looking back over the many positive results we had achieved made us both feel very humble that we could be used to show a way forward in a world where so many systems have failed. And nearly 40 years after we first met, we both agreed that nature is still our best friend.